The Clinical Thinking of W. R. Bion in Brazil

'This is an extraordinary book. These encounters with Bion and his interlocutors, followed by a rich panoply of commentaries, are thrilling, moving, sometimes funny, occasionally dangerous and deeply wise.'

Anne Alvarez, author of *The Thinking Heart* (Routledge, 2012)

'Levine, de Mattos Brito and Junqueiro de Mattos have given us an invaluable gift – an additional collection of seminars, accompanied by perceptive commentaries, which take us into the heart of Bion's clinical thinking, providing us with another vertex from which to observe the complexity of his thinking. Bion does not agree to take on the role of the one who knows, but rather takes us on an excursion through his mind, in the attempt to listen and find words for the ineffable emotional experience. Bion allows himself to be stimulated by the material presented to him, guided by his faith in the psychoanalytic method. If we agree to surrender to this way of listening, we too can be suddenly struck and moved by a new thought that dawns on us. Bion illustrates his way of working, always deeply aware of the immense difficulty in being an analyst, in finding "a language which conveys what you want it to convey, and at the same time, which the patient could understand", struggling against the perpetual "pressure to become insensitive, to grow a crust".'

Avner Bergstein, Israel Psychoanalytic Society; author of *Bion and Meltzer's Expeditions into Unmapped Mental Life* (Routledge, 2018)

'It is impossible not to be enthusiastic about this book. These fully recorded events offer readers the opportunity to follow Bion, as he expresses his ideas across 13 supervisions during his four visits to Brazil. Bion's comments reflect his evolving interest in working with the undifferentiated layers of the mind and the application of his intuitive approach. Additional layers of thought are added by the accompanying commentaries of senior Brazilian psychoanalysts, along with a precious *Introduction* by Nicola Abel-Hirsch.'

João Carlos Braga, Full Member, Supervisor, and Training Analyst at São Paulo's Brazilian Psychoanalytic Society and Psychoanalytic Group of Curitiba

The Clinical Thinking of W. R. Bion in Brazil is comprised of thirteen transcriptions of supervisions Wilfred Bion conducted during his three teaching and speaking tours of Brazil.

During these tours, Bion conducted over 130 public supervisions of analytic cases in English in which he explained his theories and illustrated their clinical application. Following on from the first volume, *Bion in Brazil: Supervisions and Commentaries* (2017), this book presents each supervision in full, with an accompanying commentary written by a senior Brazilian psychoanalyst and Bionian scholar. Arguably, no psychoanalyst has had as much impact on psychoanalytic development in Brazil than Bion, and this collection of his seminars, presented here for the first time, acts as a historical document and testament to his legacy in contemporary analysis.

The Clinical Thinking of W. R. Bion in Brazil provides a unique opportunity for contemporary psychoanalysts, candidates, and students to hear the distinctive 'voice' of Bion, observe how he listens in conversation, and learn how he would intervene in and interpret a clinical situation.

Howard B. Levine is a private practitioner in Brookline, Massachusetts, USA. He is editor-in-chief of the Routledge Wilfred R. Bion Studies Book Series, the author of *Affect, Representation and Language: Between the Silence and the Cry* (2021) and has edited and co-edited *Unrepresented States and the Construction of Meaning* (2013), *André Green Revisited: Representation and the Work of the Negative* (2018), *The Post-Bionian Field Theory of Antonino Ferro* (2021), and *The Freudian Matrix of André Green* (2023).

Gisèle de Mattos Brito is a Training and Supervising Analyst of the Psychoanalytic Society of Minas Gerais (SBPMG), Brazil, a full member of the Psychoanalytic Society of São Paulo (SBPSP), Brazil, and a former President of SBPMG. She co-edited the first volume of *Bion in Brazil* (2017) and is the author of many book chapters and scientific papers published in regional, national, and international psychoanalytic journals. Since 2009, she has coordinated the study of Bion's Supervision Seminars at the Society of São Paulo.

José Américo Junqueira de Mattos is a member and Training and Supervising Analyst of the Brazilian Society of Psychoanalysis of São Paulo and the Brazilian Society of Psychoanalysis of Ribeirão Preto. He has published many papers both in Brazil and abroad and is responsible for the preservation of Bion's Brazilian Supervisions. Since the beginning of his career, he has been interested in the ideas of Bion, who was his analyst.

The Routledge Wilfred Bion Studies Book Series
Series Editor
Howard B. Levine, MD

Editorial Advisory Board
Nicola Abel-Hirsch, Joseph Aguayo, Avner Bergstein, Lawrence J. Brown, Judith Eekhoff, Robert D. Hinshelwood, Chris Mawson, James Ogilvie, Elias M. da Rocha Barros, Jani Santamaria, Rudi Vermote

The contributions of Wilfred Bion are among the most cited in the analytic literature. Their appeal lies not only in their content and explanatory value, but in their generative potential. Although Bion's training and many of his clinical instincts were deeply rooted in the classical tradition of Freud and Melanie Klein, his ideas have a potentially universal appeal. Rather than emphasizing a particular psychic content (e.g., Oedipal conflicts in need of resolution; splits that needed to be healed; preconceived transferences that must be allowed to form and flourish, etc.), he tried to help open and prepare the mind of the analyst (without memory, desire or theoretical preconception) for the encounter with the patient.

Bion's formulations of group mentality and the psychotic and non-psychotic portions of the mind, his theory of thinking and emphasis on facing and articulating the truth of one's existence so that one might truly learn firsthand from one's own experience, his description of psychic development (alpha function and container/contained) and his exploration of **O** are 'non-denominational' concepts that defy relegation to a particular school or orientation of psychoanalysis. Consequently, his ideas have taken root in many places.... and those ideas continue to inform many different branches of psychoanalytic inquiry and interest.[1]

It is with this heritage and its promise for the future developments of psychoanalysis in mind that we present *The Routledge Wilfred Bion Studies Book Series*. This series gathers together under newly emerging and continually evolving contributions to psychoanalytic thinking that rest upon Bion's foundational texts and explore and extend the implications of his thought. For a full list of titles in the series, please visit the Routledge website at: https://www.routledge.com/The-Routledge-Wilfred-Bion-Studies-Book-Series/book-series/RWBSBS

Howard B. Levine, MD
Series Editor

---

1 Levine, H.B. and Civitarese, G. (2016). Editors' Preface, *The W.R. Bion Tradition*, Levine and Civitarese, eds., London: Karnac 2016, p. xxi.

The Clinical Thinking of W. R. Bion in Brazil

Supervisions and Commentaries

Edited by Howard B. Levine,
Gisèle de Mattos Brito, and
José Américo Junqueira de Mattos

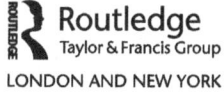
Routledge
Taylor & Francis Group

LONDON AND NEW YORK

Designed cover image: © Hilda Catz

First published 2024
by Routledge
4 Park Square, Milton Park, Abingdon, Oxon OX14 4RN

and by Routledge
605 Third Avenue, New York, NY 10158

Routledge is an imprint of the Taylor & Francis Group, an informa business

© 2024 selection and editorial matter, Howard B. Levine, Gisèle de Mattos Brito, and José Américo Junqueira de Mattos; individual chapters, the contributors

British Library Cataloguing-in-Publication Data
A catalogue record for this book is available from the British Library

Library of Congress Cataloging-in-Publication Data
Names: Levine, Howard B., editor. | Mattos Brito, Gisele de, editor. | Junqueira de Mattos, José Américo, editor.
Title: The clinical thinking of W.R. Bion in Brazil: supervisions and commentaries/edited by Howard B. Levine, Gisèle de Mattos Brito, and José Américo Junqueira de Mattos.
Description: Abingdon, Oxon; New York, NY: Routledge, 2024. | Series: The Routledge Wilfred R. Bion studies book series | Includes bibliographical references. |
Identifiers: LCCN 2023030783 (print) | LCCN 2023030784 (ebook) | ISBN 9781032553467 (paperback) | ISBN 9781032574103 (hardback) | ISBN 9781003439233 (ebook)
Subjects: LCSH: Bion, Wilfred R. (Wilfred Ruprecht), 1897-1979. | Psychoanalysis. | Psychoanalysts—Supervision of—Brazil.
Classification: LCC RC438.6.B54 C55 2024 (print) | LCC RC438.6.B54 (ebook) |
DDC 616.89/17—dc23/eng/20230921
LC record available at https://lccn.loc.gov/2023030783
LC ebook record available at https://lccn.loc.gov/2023030784

ISBN: 978-1-032-57410-3 (hbk)
ISBN: 978-1-032-55346-7 (pbk)
ISBN: 978-1-003-43923-3 (ebk)

DOI: 10.4324/9781003439233

Typeset in Times new roman
by codeMantra

Special Thanks
Gisèle and I would like to dedicate this book to her father and our co-editor, Dr. José Américo Junqueira de Mattos, without whose determination and devotion to the work of Bion, these supervisions and so much else of Bion's Brazilian legacy would not have been preserved and elaborated upon.

Howard B. Levine

Contents

Foreword

Howard B. Levine
Caveat Emptor!

It is a privilege and an enormous opportunity, one afforded us by the dedication of our colleague and co-editor, José Américo Junqueira de Mattos to preserving the thoughts and words of Bion in his Brazilian Seminars and Supervisions, that we have in our archives more than 130 of Bion's public supervisions of analytic cases. This unique treasure trove offers readers the opportunity to imaginatively experience, albeit indirectly, this extraordinary thinker as he evocatively elaborates upon his theories and illustrates how they might inform his clinical thinking and interventions.

For Bion, psychoanalytic theory and the models that it offers are a paradoxical matter. On the one hand, they are an inescapable filter through which some kind of sense might be made of the essential chaos of raw, factual existential Experience.[2] From this vertex, experience provides us with 'pre-conceptions' and an inevitable and potentially useful psychoanalytic vertex of observation in the analytic situation. On the other hand, theories and models too readily applied are a potential set of blinders that can obscure the relevant, sometimes deeply hidden singularities of the analyst's and patient's Experience, by imposing on it a false air of recognition and familiarity. It is the work of the ego to assimilate the uncanny, the strange, the unwanted, the unfamiliar in our Experience to the safety of the known. This tendency offers us a sense of anchorage and solidity in our daily existence, but it can also interfere with the stimulus to psychic growth by imprisoning us in a refuge from the pain of that necessary and desirable evolution, that Bion referred to as 'catastrophic change.'

Resounding throughout these supervisions is Bion's conviction that the 'correctness,' the presumed 'truth' or 'falsity' of psychoanalytic models and theories is a secondary matter in comparison to their potential pragmatic value of aiding and

---

2 I am using the convention of capitalizing the letter E to indicate not yet transformed, raw, existential Experience (O) and using the lower case letter e to indicate that part of Experience that we can come to know (K) and that we colloquially refer to as our 'experience.'

catalyzing psychic growth and development in the analytic situation. In Supervision D7, he says:

> *I have a kind of psychoanalytic prejudice. I have a kind of psychoanalytic preconception. Now, this prejudice leads me to suppose that there is such a thing as transference, but it's a theory. It doesn't mean that the theory is wrong, but it doesn't mean that the theory is right. It's just a theory and theories are neither right nor wrong, they may be useful or not useful.*

If readers will set this statement in an internal dialog with Bion's (1970) famous admonition to try to enter each session without memory, desire or understanding, to try to begin each moment of encounter anew and then see what it evokes as experience – and what that experience stimulates in the way of thought and feeling, conscious and unconscious – they will appreciate the complexity – and delicacy – of the analytic net that Bion would have us try to set out and that is needed to catch the most ephemeral of wild thoughts that may be present moment to moment in an analysis.

And if this was not difficult enough, once we have caught wind of something, there then follows the problem of what to say or do with or about what we may have gleaned compounded by the impossibilities and vagaries of language.

> ... ordinary language, the ordinary conversation language that we use, isn't really good enough for psychoanalysts, for psychoanalysis.
>
> (Supervision D2)

Bion insists that psychoanalysis is an *emotional experience* that takes place in the here-and-now of the analytic session within and between the analyst and analysand. He would have us empty our minds of premeditated attention (*table rosa*) so that we might better center our emergent, 'captured' attention on the emotional experience taking place. The latter is assumed to have an origin (O) that is common to both participants, even as Bion is aware that this (O) common to both participants is, at its essence and root, unknowable!

In Supervision A13, he tells us:

> ... we have to invent the language in which to interpret. What we have to interpret is what we have already seen and heard and observed in the office.

First, there is the question of finding a language that will permit the translation of the analyst's experience into thoughts and those thoughts into words. But then there is the matter of the patient. Will he or she be able to understand, tolerate and make use of that language?

> *You must talk the language that he could be able to understand, so part of it, is you and what you've learned – part of it – but the other part of it, what can he understand? What would he be likely to hear?*
>
> (Supervision A13)

Repeatedly, Bion asks his audience:

what language are you going to talk? That depends, partly, on what language you can speak yourself; but it also depends on whether the language you talk, is the kind of language, which your patient would understand. So, quite a lot is involved in this matter. You have to know what your vocabulary is and what your language is and what language and vocabulary, your patient would understand.
(Supervision A13)

Systematically, Bion emphasizes the great difficulty of putting into words the lived experience of the moment and transmitting it.

Now, as a matter of fact, the kind of thinking and the kind of talking that we do in analysis is not ordinary talking, it's not even about an ordinary subject; so, it can be very difficult for the patient to know that she doesn't know much about psychoanalysis or, for that matter, about thinking.
(Supervision A49)

as analysts, we have to invent the tools we use, as we are using them. It sounds easy, because it sounds as if we just use the ordinary language. Well, so we do, but we don't mean quite the same ordinary things. That's the trouble.
(Supervision D2)

But this trouble is what we might call 'good trouble,' as it is the potential stimulus to creativity, thought and psychic development in both analysand and analyst.

Having forewarned – and perhaps forearmed – the reader, I will leave you here and in the spirit of Bion ask you to try to empty your minds as you begin to experience this book and see what you can make of it, what it will make of you and where it will lead you to.

Authors' bios

Nicola Abel-Hirsch is a Training and Supervising Analyst of the British Psychoanalytic Society and works in private practice in London. She has given clinical and theoretical seminars and papers on Bion in the UK, Taiwan, the USA and Europe. From 2013 to 2015 she was Visiting Professor at the University of Essex' Centre for Psychoanalytic Studies. She is the author of many psychoanalytic papers and the book, *Bion: 365 Quotes* (2019), and the editor of Hanna Segal's last book, *Yesterday, Today and Tomorrow* (2007).

Deocleciano Bendocchi Alves is a medical doctor and holds a degree in the theoretical and practical psychoanalysis of adults, children and adolescents from the São Paulo Institute of Psychoanalysis. He is a Training Analyst of the Brazilian Society of Psychoanalysis of São Paulo. He leads study groups on Bion's *Cogitations* and *Memoir of Future* and has published many papers on clinical psychoanalysis. He attended courses, seminars, supervisions and conferences given by W.R. Bion in Brazil in 1974, 1975 and 1978.

Altamirando M. Andrade Jr. is Past President, Director of Training, Supervisor and Training Analyst and Member of the Faculty of the Brazilian Psychoanalytic Society of Rio de Janeiro (SBPRJ). He was Latin American Representative to the Board of the IPA (2011-2015) and has been Chair of the IPA Ethics Committee since 2016.

José Renato Avzaradel is a Training and Supervising Analyst of the Brazilian Psychoanalytic Society of Rio de Janeiro, a member of the IPA's Inter-Regional Encyclopedic Dictionary Task Force, has edited and co-edited books *About Language and Thinking* (2012) and *Language and the Construction of Thinking* (2005) and has published papers in the IJP, the RBP and the Annual of Psychoanalysis.

Marli Claudete Braga is a graduate in Psychology from the Catholic University of Paraná, in Philosophy from the Federal University of Paraná and in child and adolescent psychoanalysis from the Psychoanalytic Society of São Paulo. She is a member of the IPA, the Brazilian Psychoanalytic Society of São Paulo, the

Brazilian Psychoanalytic Society of Rio de Janeiro and the Curitiba Psychoanalytic Group, where she is also a Training Analyst.

Gisèle de Mattos Brito is a Training and Supervising Analyst of the Psychoanalytic Society of Minas Gerais (SBPMG), Brasil, a full member of the Psychoanalytic Society of São Paulo (SBPSP), Brasil and a former President of SBPMG. She co-edited the first volume of Bion in Brazil (Karnac, 2017) and is the author of many book chapters and scientific papers published in regional, national and international psychoanalytic journals. Since 2009, she has coordinated the study of Bion's Supervision Seminars at the Society of São Paulo.

Celso Antonio Vieira de Camargo is a full member of the Brazilian Society of Psychoanalysis of São Paulo, was an Assistant Professor at São Marcos Faculdade de Filosofia, Psicologia e Ciência de Letras in 1975–1976, worked as a Psychiatrist and Chief of Staff in a Psychiatric Hospital from 1976 to 1978, and is now in private practice. He was associate editor of the "Jornal de Psicanálise," 2017–2018 and helped organize the twelve Psicanálise:Bion Encounters in Brazil.

Claudio Castelo Filho is a full member and Training Analyst at the Sociedade Brasileira de Psicanálise de São Paulo, Brazil, where he is in private practice. He holds a Master's Degree in Clinical Psychology from Pontifícia Universidade Católica de São Paulo, a PhD in Social Psychology and is Professor of Clinical Psychology at the Universidade de São Paulo. He is a full member of the International Psychoanalytical Association (IPA) and the Federação de Psicanálise da América Latina (FEPAL), the author of the books *O Processo Criativo: Transformação e Ruptura* (São Paulo, Blucher, 2015), *A Psicanálise do Vir a Ser* (Blucher, São Paulo, 2020) and organizer and author of the book *Sobre o Feminino* (Blucher, São Paulo, 2018). He has published widely in Brazil, Italy and the USA (On the Verge of 'Madness'; Creativity and the Fear of Insanity, in *Explorations in Bion's 'O,'* New York, Routledge, 2019) and is also a painter with exhibitions and publications in Brazil, Germany and England.

Juarez Guedes Cruz is a Training and Supervising Analyst at the Psychoanalytical Society of Porto Alegre. In addition to psychoanalytical publications, he is the author of three books of short stories: *The Chronology of Gestures'* (Movimento Editor, 2003, Porto Alegre) – winner of the Açorianos Award, 2004, *Some Procedures to Hide Wounds* (Movimento Editor, 2007, Porto Alegre) and *Before Mirrors Become Opaque* (Dublinense Editor, 2012, Porto Alegre). In 2007, he edited an anthology of short stories entitled *Paradox of Tchekov* (Nova Prova Editor, 2007, Porto Alegre).

Aldo Luiz Duarte graduated as a psychiatrist from the Federal University of Rio Grande do Sul (Universidade Federal do Rio Grande do Sul), Brazil, is a graduate candidate at the Institute of Psychoanalysis of the Psychoanalytic Society of Porto Alegre (Sociedade Psicanalítica de Porto Alegre), Brazil and a Psychoanalytic Psychotherapy Supervisor at the Psychiatry Residency of the St. Peter Psychiatric Hospital/ Department of Health of the State of Rio Grande do Sul (Hospital Psiquiátrico São Pedro/Secretaria Estadual da Saúde do Rio Grande do Sul), Brazil.

Marta Foster is a Member of the International Psychoanalytical Association and a Training and Supervising Analyst of the Brazilian Society of Psychoanalysis of São Paulo. She is the Coordinator of the "Analysts' Professional Development" and the "Masterpieces of Sigmund Freud and Wilfred Bion" Study Groups at the Brazilian Society of Psychoanalysis of São Paulo. Her scientific articles have been published in the *Brazilian Psychoanalytic Journal*, the *Brazilian Psychoanalysis Magazine* and in the book *Researching with the Psychoanalytical Method* edited by Escuta.

José Américo Junqueira de Mattos graduated from the Institute of Psychoanalysis of the Brazilian Society of psychoanalysis of São Paulo. He was one of the five founding members of the Psychoanalysis Group that later became the Brazilian Society of Psychoanalysis of Ribeirão Preto and has been a Training Analyst in both Societies. He has published several papers published both in Brazil and abroad. Since the beginning of his career he has been interested in the ideas of Bion, who was his analyst.

Howard B. Levine is a member of APSA, PINE, the Contemporary Freudian Society, Pulsion, on the faculty of NYU Post-Doc's Contemporary Freudian Track, on the Editorial Board of the IJP and Psychoanalytic Inquiry, editor-in-chief of the *Routledge Wilfred Bion Studies Book Series* and in private practice in Brookline, Massachusetts. He is the author of *Transformations de l'Irreprésentable* (Ithaque, 2019) and *Affect, Representation and Language: Between the Silence and the Cry* (Routledge, 2022) and editor of *The Post-Bionian Field Theory of Antonino Ferro* (Routledge, 2022) and *The Freudian Matrix of Andre Green. Towards A Psychoanalysis For The 21st Century* by André Green (Routledge/IPA, 2023). His co-edited books include *Unrepresented States and the Construction of Meaning* (Karnac, 2013); *On Freud's Screen Memories* (Karnac, 2014); *The Wilfred Bion Tradition* (Karnac, 2016); *Bion in Brazil vol.1* (Karnac, 2017); *Andre Green Revisited: Representation and the Work of the Negative* (Karnac, 2018); *Covidian Life* (Phoenix, 2021); *Psychoanalysis of the Psychoanalytic Frame Revisited: A New Look at Bleger's Classical Work* (Routledge/IPA, 2022) and *Autistic Phenomena and Unrepresented States: Explorations in the Emergence of Self* (Phoenix, 2023).

Ruggero Levy is a Training and Supervising Analyst at the Psychoanalytic Society from Porto Alegre (SPPA), Brasil, a former President of SPPA and former Director of the SPPA's Institute of Psychoanalysis. He is Chair of the IPA Working Parties Committee, ex-IPA Board Member from 2011 to 2015, Professor and supervisor of the Federal University of Rio Grande do Sul in Child, Adolescent and Adult Psychotherapy and author of many book chapters and scientific papers published in regional, national and international psychoanalytic journals and reviews.

Evelise de Souza Marra is a Training and Supervising Analyst at the Psychoanalytic Society of São Paulo (SBPSP). She holds bachelor's and master's degrees in psychology from the University of São Paulo and has taught psychoanalysis and couples' therapy at the Catholic University of São Paulo for sixteen years.

Cecil José Rezze is a seminar leader and Training and Supervising Analyst at the Psychoanalysis Institute of Sao Paulo (SBPSP). He received his PhD from the Medical School of the University of São Paulo, was Editor-in-Chief of *Revista Brasileira de Psicanálise* (1977/1978), past President of SBPSP (1979/1980), Co-chair, of the I-XIII Annual Bion Psychoanalytic Meetings (2008 to 2021) and has presented and published at many congresses, journals and books.

Introduction

A route into the supervisions

Nicola Abel-Hirsch

My aim has been to draw out what the different supervisions have in common in order to offer the reader some signposts in approaching them.

OUTLINE

1 Beginnings: general descriptions will not suffice, Bion wants the details of who thought what and what exactly was said.
2 Bion often then goes on to change the vertex from which the material is viewed.
3 At the centre of the supervisions is a focus on the transference.
4 The authority of the analyst and the respect for the patient
5 Observation and Intuition
6 On some differences between these supervisions and those given three years earlier in 1975.

1. Beginnings: general descriptions will not suffice, Bion wants the details of who thought what and what exactly was said

As little as possible is to be taken for granted. When general remarks are made by the presenting analyst in their introduction, Bion asks for specifics, including in this any underlying relationships that may be affecting the case, i.e. Did you know the previous analyst? He makes it clear that there isn't only one description of the realities of the beginning of an analysis, but each person has their own point of view or vertex [Bion's preferred term]. His attempt to find out the detail is often happening amidst a chaos of noise and the difficulties of translation. He is encouraging, "yes, yes!" being his frequent response. Some examples:

Chapter 6

Bion: Did he tell you that he had had analysis before?
A: Yes. He did.
Bion: Yes! Did you say anything about that? Did you reply, interpret it to him?

DOI: 10.4324/9781003439233-1

Chapter 10

Bion: Who had said that the patient was a psychotic?

[The seminar struggles with the question]

> *I think that the question being answered is a much more difficult one than I'm asking. I'll put it this way: whose idea was it that he was ill or wanted help?*

Bion: *Why I'm asking the question is: where does the idea come from that this patient needs help? Now, we can understand what the analyst and so on did. But the interesting thing is that apparently the patient thinks he needs help. In other words, he's not so mad that he doesn't know that he needs help. There are plenty of people who can be what we call insane, but wouldn't want any help from anybody. They could feel that they were quite all right; but this patient seems, at any rate, to be sufficiently well to know that he's ill.*

Chapter 11

> *She had a man as a psychoanalyst.*

Bion: Did you know the psychoanalyst?

2. A change of vertex

Having established something of who actually said and did what, Bion changes the vertex and provides an often radically different view of the presenting material. Some examples:

Chapter 2

In Chapter 2, we hear from the presenting analyst that the patient: "feels like his anus and rectum would be open and he is waiting for the entering of something – a penis for instance". Bion checks if it is the patient who has said this and after further discussion he comments:

Bion: *Yes, but what strikes me about it is; I'm quite prepared to believe he has this irritation in his penis and that orifice is wide open. After all, the patient ought to know – I have a particular reason to believe he's trying to tell me lies, although he may not be. But, what I wonder is: what's happened to all the other orifices? What about the other end of the alimentary canal? What about the mouth? What about the ears? Are they shut to interpretations? Why only that orifice?*

Bion goes beyond the content of what the patient has said and looks at his behaviour in the session. It seems the patient is taking in little of what the analyst says to him. Instead of looking downwards towards the penis, Bion then metaphorically turns around and looks up the alimentary canal to the mouth and ears.

Chapter 5

In the supervision in Chapter 5 Bion presents one of his own cases. He tells us that the patient talked 'quite freely' and came to every session. He was rational and co-operative, and never ill, not even a cold. The patient had some bother getting on the couch, but not enough to initially catch Bion's attention.

> *Bion: I thought that I would change my vertex, because I thought that I obviously couldn't see anything very much from where I was looking or observing this patient. But, when I did that, it occurred to me that his precise and exact position on the couch could be comprehensible if he were lying of the edge of a precipice and then, his position, his posture, began to look very much like a cataleptic attitude and the whole analysis began to look like a sort of compulsive ritual....*
>
> *The total situation in the consulting room could be a "follies a deux"....*
>
> *Then, I began to look at and listen to the behaviour of both these people, one of whom was myself!*

Looked at from the first vertex the analysis is proceeding cooperatively. When Bion changes his vertex, he sees the patient on the couch lying as if "on the edge of a precipice" and himself and the patient in a "follies a deux" [the sharing of delusional ideas by two people who are closely associated].

Chapter 8

The patient is feeling guilty about not going to another town to take care of her dying father. Bion is concerned that the presenting analyst's interpretation could sound as if he were saying the patient should devote herself to her parents. Bion changes the vertex and turns our view of the Oedipus complex on its head. 'Oedipus' is now guilty about not bringing up his father and not marrying his mother!

Bion: *The difficulty I see about this is: how to give such an interpretation, because, if you say something of that sort, then, it sounds to the patient, exactly as if, in your opinion, you thought that the patient should devote themselves to the parents, which isn't what one wants to say. What one wants to do is: to draw attention to the guilt there is about the fact that one does not bring up one's father or mother, one does not marry one's father, nor does one marry one's mother; but, for some reason, the universe isn't made like that. It's not made like that in the first instance and in the present, there are other things which the person concerned has to do.*

Some background to Bion's use of a change of vertex

In addition to his natural capacity to make such unexpected changes of view, Bion has consciously and intentionally been employing this method since at least his group-work in the 1940s (*Experiences in Groups* published in 1961). In the following quote from this period, he talks about altering his focus rather as one might alter the focus of a microscope.

> *I am reminded of looking through a microscope at an over thick section; with one focus I see, not very clearly perhaps, but with sufficient distinctness, one picture. If I alter the focus very slightly I see another. Using this as an analogy for what I am doing mentally, I shall now have another look at this group, and will then describe the pattern that I see with the altered focus.*
>
> *The picture of hard-working individuals striving to solve their psychological problems is displaced by a picture of a group mobilized to express its hostility and contempt for neurotic patients and for all who may wish to approach neurotic problems seriously. This group at the moment seems to me to be led by the two absentees, who are indicating that there are better ways of spending their time than by engaging in the sort of experience with which the group is familiar when I am a member of it. At a previous session this group was led by one of the members now absent.*
>
> (CWB IV, pp. 136–137)

It is a method that Bion continued to use. Here is another example from some twenty years later. In what he calls a psychoanalytic game, Bion suggests that the analyst might take an interpretation he has been satisfied with, and put it into Col. 2 of the Grid [statements being used defensively] and then ask him or herself what the interpretation, correct though it may be, might be excluding. He interestingly also comments that this can be a way of exercising and developing one's capacity for intuition.

> *The analyst can set himself similar exercises not as a mere tax on his ingenuity, but as a method of exercising and developing his capacity for intuition.*
>
> (*Elements* 1963 CWB V, p. 114)

3. At the centre of the supervisions is a focus on the transference

I was surprised to find just how much Bion talks about the transference. I think that in these supervisions we see something terribly important about how he puts together the work he has done on 'being in' rather than 'knowing about' analysis/oneself, with working in the transference. Working in the transference involves leaving one's private life out of it [see Chapter 1 below]. It involves always attending to how one is being experienced by the patient. By leaving his or her idiosyncratic individual self out of the picture, the analyst can be more present. Some examples:

Chapter 1

The supervision begins with the presenting analyst describing his patient waiting for him in the corridor when he [the analyst] is five minutes late. The patient comments on his lateness and on another change from the usual course of events and suggests that something has changed in the analyst's practice. Bion comes in immediately with the following comment:

Bion: *Yes. I'd like to take up this point for a moment. One of the reasons for not telling the patients anything about one's own private life, or difficulties and so on is: it stimulates ideas in the patient which may not be, at all, important. Now, if I don't tell the patient anything about my private life, it's not because I've got anything to hide particularly. I don't really mind very much, because in any case, people hear about the analyst – in any community, there's a great deal of talk – but I don't tell anything, because it leaves them more space in which to use their imagination.*

In the analysis it doesn't matter what I think, or who I am, or what my troubles are. That is a matter of absolute unimportance. The only thing which is important in the analysis is the patient's thoughts, the patient's ideas, the patient's feelings.

Bion comments that the patient can, of course, 'analyse' him. He doesn't want to stop that and couldn't even if he wanted to.

In the same way, this patient can hear all sorts of things about the analyst, but none of it is of any importance. What is important is what that patient thinks – independent of whether those thoughts are factually right or wrong. So, from this point of view, while one can interpret: *"You are feeling that I think this"*, or *"I think that"*, or *"I think the other"*, that isn't because I am important, but because *the patient* thinks it – that's what makes it important. So, you could say about this:

Yes, I can see that you think that I'm late and I have changed and so on… That doesn't very much matter if that is true; it doesn't much matter if it's untrue, but what is important is that you, the patient, think and what you've just been telling me what happens here. The important thing here is what you think and who you are.

After some discussion and attempted clarification on the part of the translator the presenter talks about an incident two years earlier. When his daughter was born, he had phoned a patient to say he couldn't see her. She had told him recently that something important must have happened. "Perhaps it was the way that I spoke on the telephone" comments the analyst. The analyst I think may want to say that ordinary human contact between patient and analyst is important. Bion however continues to think about the transference with the first patient:

> *Now, what age is this character who thinks that the analyst is and behaves as if the analyst was a very important person and that this very important person can spend time looking at him as if he were a very important person? What age is he? The physical fact of his being thirtyeight we needn't bother with it, because it would be no good telling him that he is thirtyeight. He knows all that. So, the one question would be: what age is this person, who thinks that you are a very important person and that you, a very important person, is bothering about him, as if he were a very important person?*

Chapter 7

Bion listens for the most primitive transference he can hear to be occurring between the presenting analyst and his or her patient. In this example it is of an infant's experience of coming up against an object that doesn't have a breast.

Bion: *One has to think of it in terms, again, that it sounds very primitive. It sounds as if it really is on that kind of breast feeding level, this wild animal and so forth... Now, a baby, I think, doesn't really make much difference between a father and a mother – not at first. So that, the baby expects to be put to the breast whether it's by the father or the mother. So, when it begins to find that the father does not behave like the mother, presses out towards this object and instead of finding it, getting a breast, it gets something else. So, I think that in this respect, probably, you are much more the person who does not put her to the breast. All that you do is: just talk. It's difficult to say, because, that's what everybody expects, analysis is only talk; nevertheless, if she is expecting to get something good, such as an infant might experience if it were put to the breast, then, it is a very great shock.*

As with the history referred to above of his changing the vertex from his group work in the 1940s [and probably all his life], Bion also has a long history of addressing what he thinks could be the infantile transference in an adult psychoanalysis. The best known example is perhaps that in 'On Arrogance' (1958) when he constructs a picture of the patient as an infant whose has been refused his mother's containment.

Chapter 9

Chapter 9 is particularly rich in his descriptions and discussions of the patient's effect on the analyst in the transference. We tend to refer to this as the analyst's countertransference. Bion, however, stresses that the countertransference is unconscious and I don't think he would call this the countertransference. See, for example, Chapter 4.

Bion: *No, it doesn't matter! There is nothing that the analyst can do about counter-transference.*

In Chapter 9 Bion is in fact talking about what we today call enactment. He wants to help people have the necessary tools to sustain the analytic position [to continue to be able to think].

Bion: *Anyhow, suppose it was a surgical operation. It doesn't help the surgical operation if the surgeon is interrupted in such a way that he can't operate properly. Similarly, it's not a good thing if the analyst is made to have such strong feelings that he can't think clearly. It's not that we want to be like computers ... But we try not to make too big mistakes, because then it becomes difficult to think clearly. ... We would like to be able to be just ordinary people trying to do ... to help – that's all we're trying to do, anyway.*

So, even if the patient is trying to make you angry, or to control the situation by making you fall in love, or something of that kind, one doesn't resist it to frustrate the patient, but simply, because one does not think so clearly when one is dominated by feelings of fear, or love, or hate, of the patient....

...I try, if I can, when I'm talking English, to avoid terms like: sadism or masochism, but to use something like: "You like being cruel!" or "You like being cruelly treated, you're wanting me to say something cruel to you!" That's why patients, sometimes, try to make the analyst angry, partly because he knows that analysts don't want to be angry, so he can get the pleasure of making the analyst feel and behave in a way in which the analyst does not want to feel or behave. In that very situation, again, you can get the pleasure of making the analyst feel what he doesn't want to feel and getting yourself the pleasure of being angrily treated, cruelly treated.

Chapter 13

Bion's focus understandably leads to his being asked if everything in the relationship between patient and analyst is "always based on transference". He answers:

Bion: *... the real point about transference is that it's only a psychoanalytic theory of a link between two people, it's talking about a relationship....*

And sometime later in the seminar, Bion makes the following comment:

Bion: *Well, I'll put it a little bit differently because I would say that I have a kind*
          of psychoanalytic prejudice. I have a kind of psychoanalytic preconcep-
          tion. Now, this prejudice leads me to suppose that there is such a thing as
          transference, but it's a theory. It doesn't mean that the theory is wrong, but
          it doesn't mean that the theory is right. It's just a theory and theories are
          neither right nor wrong, they may be useful or not useful.

To my knowledge Bion doesn't address the question of what else the relationship
between patient and analyst could be based on [i.e. the aspect of the relationship
that is described in some psychoanalytic orientations as the working alliance, or the
earlier question about its including simple human contact]. Instead, he addresses
some of what it means to look at the link between patient and analyst through the
lens of the theory of transference. He doesn't want to give a didactic account of
the transference. I think he wants to keep sight of just how much we do not know.
The use of the theory of transference, he says, inevitably prejudices what he understands. At the same time, he is referring to the potential operation of theory at
the deep level of a preconception. By the use of the term preconception, we have a
view of theory in intimate contact with its realization in the experience of the session. The psychoanalyst Dennis Duncan puts it thus:

> *When an analyst has found his way to a theoretical construct which speaks for*
> *him the inner experience of his sessions, and when a theory has symbolically*
> *entered that experience, it has a meaningfulness and instrumentality which is*
> *not conveyed in the face-value theoretical statement.*
>
> (Duncan 1981 p. 347)

Bion is intending to talk about the use of theory at the level of being an analyst, not
its use to 'know about analysis'.

In the same seminar the participants persevere in their questioning Bion about
the place he is according the transference. Does he ever not use the transference?

P1:   May I ask you a personal question?
Bion: Yes!
P1:   *Do you sometimes work in a different way, different from the classical way*
          – not using transference, for example, in some situations?
Bion: *I depart from it with extreme reluctance and don't like doing so. I don't*
          think it's good enough, but I don't know anything better, but I'm sure it isn't
          good enough....
Bion: *Yes. Now, I also want to suggest that as well as this, there is sensuous,*
          infra-sensuous and ultra-sensuous, and this space has got to be increased
          to provide the room for the analyst who's seeing a schizophrenic patient.
P1:   You call the space?...
Bion: *Umhm... I think that the... I'd like to change the words a bit and say: the*
          human animal, like all animal life, does not like the unknown. So, when

confronted with the unknown, the human animal, like all other animals, has both curiosity and fear stimulated and you've got this situation in which curiosity has to be exercised, while the person is afraid ...

Work in the transference does not make it an as-if or intellectual encounter between analyst and patient. Bion stresses the requirement to be more open to the patient than we may be familiar with, and that analytic work confronts us with a frightening unknown.

4. The authority of the analyst and respect for the patient

Bion is concerned in the supervisions to draw out the difference between being more open to the unknown and loosening one's authority as analyst. Participants also sometimes confuse being available to the patient with allowing the patient to denigrate them. Some examples:

Chapter 2: The authority of the analyst

Bion: *...What is an analyst to tell a patient, who already knows all the answers? You'll often get a patient who either goes on talking as if they hadn't heard what you'd said or else, whatever the analyst says: "yes, I know. Yes, I know". They brush aside the interpretation, because they know all the answers. So, there's no room to learn anything. That doesn't mean to say that the analyst is wrong. It's quite a difficult problem what to say next when the patient says: "yes I know"; actually, it's very much the same when the patient says: "I don't know what you're talking about", it's tempting to reply: "I know you don't" or "since you know everything, it's no good going on with it". But, I think that one has to resist that temptation, and nevertheless, persist with whatever things one can say or do.*

Chapter 3: The authority of the analyst

Bion: *...Because of this intensity, because of the power of the matter we're talking about, it's difficult to point out that in talking about certain things, we take these matters very seriously. That's why we think it's worth spending so much time and money over it. But patients very often don't believe that we know what they're talking about. So, you're sure to have to say it over and over again.*

Chapter 7: Respect for the patient, Why is the patient coming for analysis?

A: *...Do you remember that last week, you asked, many times, why this patient was coming to me.*

Bion: *Um hum.*

A: *It's not an answer, but one thing I am thinking is that she knows me since some years ago, when I did the seminars about "Baby Observation".*

Bion: *Yes, yes! This question as to why she comes to you is not simply a question of the first session; it crops up over and over again. Next time, you can ask yourself again: why today? Why has she come again, today? It's probably something...*

[here it's impossible to make out the word].

...it's probably because she thinks you would know what to say, or to do either: about this wild beast behavior in the son, or her own behavior, like a wild beast; but, one needn't bother about that very much, the really important thing is: the patient comes to you because she has some... Hope you see, that you will know how to deal with it.

Bion: *That statement can also be a statement of her idea of that's why you come. That you only see her because you've got nothing else to do and so on... not because you're interested in her or her family, that's her fear. So, the point about this is patients very often think: well, it's natural for you to see them, it's your profession and you earn a living that way and you're a psychologist or a psychoanalyst and she probably gets this idea from psychologists. So, she can be afraid that if you spoke the truth about it, you'd have to admit you don't really want to see her, at all.*

So that, in this matter, it's very difficult to come to you and tell you what her troubles are as if you were a friend of hers, as if you were friendly disposed. She hopes that you are, that's how she's got there so far. But, I think that if you can, you should draw her attention to the fact that she is afraid that as well as her not wanting to come and so forth... one is not saying that she wants to come, she's afraid that you don't want to come either; whether you are felt to be a sort of a mother, or husband, or wife there's still the anxiety that she might want to come to you, but you mightn't want to see her.

On other occasions the participants are more baffled. Does Bion mean patients should be able to say why they are coming? Even that analysts should ask their patients this? In some instances, Bion wants to draw attention to the fact that although the patient is dismissive of analysis they are, at the same time, coming to their session. He says he himself might challenge a patient with this observation.

In general, it is I think his intention to challenge what back in his 1940s group work he called basic assumption Dependency (baD) and to do this in relation to both the participants and their patients. It may be thought that only the more well patients can be given a more self-determining responsibility for what they do. This would not be correct because what Bion is challenging is not to do with what an individual patient needs. He is challenging a state of mind that denies the need for work and development. One of his own patients, Francis Tustin [well known for her own work on autistic states], puts it well:

Dr. Bion aroused in me the courage to see things from a different perspective from the current and accepted ones, and also different from his. He provoked me to think for myself—to have a mind of my own. He did this by asking challenging questions and by making unexpected remarks rather than by imposing a rigid interpretive scheme on what I said and did. In so doing, he made me think about what was happening to me in my own terms.

(Tustin 1981 pp. 175/176)

5. Observation and intuition

In his novel *A Memoir of the Future,* written in a few years earlier in the early 1970s, Bion makes reference to his having suffered a loss of confidence in psychoanalysis and to what then led him to persist with it. He puts observation at the centre:

Roland: What led you to persist [in being a psychoanalyst when he had doubts about its efficacy]?

P.A.[psycho-analyst]: Partly a chance recapitulation of Freud's description of the impression created on him by Charcot's insistence on continued observation of facts – unexplained facts – until a pattern began to emerge; ...

(1977 CWB XIV, p. 122)

The supervisions bear testimony to his capacity for observation and he conveys how difficult and subtle a task observation is. Here is an example:

Chapter 8: Observation

A: *The same patient. One day when she was speaking about the crystal, that she would like something in analysis like a crystal. I said something about she had edges – the crystal has edges. She protested and said: "But I am not speaking about the edges, I am speaking about the crystal, the infinite".*

Bion: *No, I was meaning in what way would you say...*
A: *That she was different?*
Bion: *Yes, because, this is the sort of thing, which is so difficult to describe.*
A: *Yes.*
Bion: *I'm asking you the question... I'm well aware that the demands on verbal expression are tremendous....*
Bion: *Yes. I think it's simply one of these things it's worth asking you the question, because, I think, it's a question which exists; you may be able to answer it, or you may be able to answer it later on, especially if you can contrast it with this more ragged worn sort of woman, on one occasion, this is a different one. So you could if there were two sisters, you might be able to compare the two, but at least...*
         [Someone coughs while Dr. Bion was speaking, blurring two or three words]
         it might be useful, if not on this occasion, on some other occasion to say what the difference is. However, I think that you make it clearer to me,

perhaps you can verbalize it yourself later on... I don't know. It really, in a sense, sounds almost more human, not so much the hard edges and the lines of the crystal, that sort of thing... (8)

Chapter 5: Intuition

The participants want to get Bion to talk about 'memory and desire', intuition and 'thoughts without a thinker'. Rather than talk about these things he invites them to participate in actually being more intuitive:

P1   *... memory and... memory and...*
P2   *Intuition!*
P1   *Intuition, and what do you think about the thought without the thinker?*
Bion: *To take the last point first, I would suggest that we imagine that when a number of people collect together, like this, there are stray thoughts float-ing around**, trying to find a mind to settle in. So, the problem from the point of each individual – one of us – is: can we catch one of these wild thoughts without being too particular about what race they are or what category they are? Whether they are memories or intuitions! But, just get hold of any one of these wild thoughts however strange or however savage or friendly they might be. Give it a home and then allow it to escape from your lungs in other words give it birth. So that, here no matter how wild the idea may be.*

6. On some differences between these supervisions and those given three years earlier (1975) and published in The complete works of Bion (2014)

Shortly before writing this chapter, I had written a chapter for another book on Bion's 1975 supervisions [supervisions that happened three years before the super-visions in this book]. I am struck by the fact that there do seem to be some differ-ences. In 1975 Bion mostly begins his contributions by questioning an assumption being made by the presenter. In the present supervisions he spends more time first trying to get an accurate picture of what is being presented. In the 1975 supervi-sions, the core of the supervisions was Bion's formulation of the patient's object relations through attending to the relationship with the analyst, the patients internal object relations, and their relationships with people in their world. In the present supervisions Bion doesn't do this anywhere near as much. Instead, he throws a closer light on how to work in the transference and how to sustain one's analytic position. The present supervisions I think have more in them about how to actually do analysis. This is invaluable.

In one of the present supervisions Bion also does something that is very unusual for him. He recounts an interpretation given to him by Klein when he was her pa-tient. Over the years he has said very very little about the content of his analyses with Rickman and Klein and yet he does so in Chapter 5. I think it may show his determination to be with the participants in the difficulties and vulnerabilities of the depth of the analytic task. I wonder too if he might be curious about the interpretation and what the participants might say about it. Here it is:

> *Now Melanie Klein gave me an interpretation which puzzled me for a long time she said: "You feel mutilated castrated, as you emerge from the womb" (Chapter 5).*

One does wonder if he connects this with all the work he is doing on allowing the emergence of what he calls "wild ideas"!

Bibliography

Bion, W. (1961). *Experiences in Groups*, CWB, volume IV.
———— (1963). *Elements of Psycho-analysis*, CWB, volume V.
———— (1977). *A Memoir of the Future Book 3: The Dawn of Oblivion*, CWB, volume XIV
———— (2014). *The Complete Works of W. R. Bion*, Editor C. Mawson, Great Britain Karnac books.
Duncan, D. (1981). A Thought on the Nature of Psychoanalytic Theory. *International Journal of Psychoanalysis*, 62:339–349.
Tustin, F. (1981). In Memoriam W. R. Bion. A Modern Pilgrim's Progress: Reminiscences of Personal Analysis with Dr. Bion. Journal of Child Psychotherapy, 7(2):175–179.

Chapter 1[1]

Supervision A13

T: He's already spoken about this client.[2] He's a thirty-eight-year-old man, this session he's bringing now is a recent session. The analyst had arrived five minutes late. The patient, who was already waiting for him in the corridor, starts straight away making comments about the analyst's being late; that he could see that something was changed in the analyst's practice, because one of his clients, apparently, had not gone to the session. He says that he was used to always being received by his analyst on time and having a client before him.

Bion: Yes. I'd like to take up this point for a moment. One of the reasons for not telling the patients anything about one's own private life, or difficulties and so on is: it stimulates ideas in the patient which may not be, at all, important. Now, if I don't tell the patient anything about my private life, it's not because I've got anything to hide particularly. I don't really mind very much, because in any case, people hear about the analyst – in any community, there's a great deal of talk – but I don't tell anything, because it leaves them more space in which to use their imagination.

In the analysis it doesn't matter what I think, or who I am, or what my troubles are. That is a matter of absolute unimportance. The only thing which is important in the analysis is the patient's thoughts, the patient's ideas, the patient's feelings. That is why I would like to keep myself out of it. I can't, of course, because the patients can analyze me, just as much as I can analyze them. I don't mind that and I don't want to stop it – I couldn't if I wanted to!

In the same way, this patient can hear all sorts of things about the analyst, but none of it is of any importance. What is important is what that patient thinks – whether it is right or wrong. So, from this point of view, while one can interpret: *"You are feeling that I think this"*, or *"I think that"*, or *"I think the other"*, that isn't because I am important, but because *the patient* thinks it – that's what makes it important. So, you could say about this:

DOI: 10.4324/9781003439233-2

Yes, I can see that you think that I'm late and I have changed and so on... That doesn't very much matter if that is true; it doesn't much matter if it's untrue, but what is important is that you, the patient, think and what you've just been telling me what happens here. The important thing here is what you think and who you are.

Now, we don't mean that therefore the patient is important – that's up to him. He can make up his own mind about that as well. But why we do this, is because we think that the individual matters. In analysis, rightly or wrongly, we think that people matter – we think that what the patient thinks matters to him.

That's why we're not talking about what I think, what we, the analysts, think. What we are concerned with is what you, the patient, thinks and feels. So all that you've heard about me and know about me, is entirely your own affair, but it doesn't matter whether I'm that person or not.

What matters to the patient is whether what he thinks is accurate or not accurate. I mention this point, because it's very liable to be distracting to be told, that you are late and that your patient is this, or your patient left you, or your patient didn't come, but, in fact, those facts in so far as they are true don't really matter. So, in this instance, for example, you could say:

You're spending so much time on this, that you must think that I'm a very important person; or else, there's a problem, as to why you spend so much time on a person who is so unimportant, as myself? If I'm really important and you think so, well, that's alright. But if I'm not really important and you think so, then it becomes important as to why you should think so. Why you think that I'm important or not important? I'm only your analyst. But since you're spending so much time talking about me, you must think that I am very important; or else, you want to know why you've been wasting your time.

T: But this is the way that the patient behaves.
Bion: The way that the patient behaves gives us a clue as to who he is.
T: I didn't translate correctly. He (A) said: *"That's the way the patient is being".*
Bion: Yes. In analysis, in your office, in your consulting room, happenings take place and they matter. Included in these happenings, are the patient's talking; but it's only *one* of the happenings.
P1:   But perhaps there's a problem about the link. He (A) said that this patient was already brought here. Could it be possible that something that

happened here that affected and was noticed by his patient?[3] Two years ago when my daughter was born, I phoned a patient saying that I could not see her. Well, the other day she told me that something very important must have happened to me then. Perhaps it was the way that I spoke on the telephone.

Bion: Why should it be very important? That's different. That tells you something about the patient. It doesn't tell the patient anything about you because, in fact, we are not important people, therefore, what in fact happens to us is a matter of no importance. It is not a matter of any importance if I got ill, or I got knocked down and killed, or had some trouble or other... That's not important. What's important in the analytic consultation is that the patient *thinks* it's important. The patient says something important must have happened – not at all! It's important because the patient thinks the analyst is important, because the patient thinks it's important what happens to his or her analyst. In fact, it's of no importance whatever because we are only ordinary human beings, we are not people of any importance.

P2:   But human beings are important!

Bion: Only to us, only to us.

P2:   But they are!

Bion: But not to anything else. An earthquake can take place, the weather can change, we can get struck by lightning, we can get struck by a disease. None of these things bother about mere insignificant creatures like us. It's only we who say: "*Homo sapiens*" and possibly one or two animals like your dog or your cat that might think it was "*Homo sapiens*"; I doubt it, but perhaps they do! But, if a gonococcus, for example – thinks at all – it might think that a human being is quite useful, but it wouldn't mind two pence if we were very wise, or stupid, or articulate or anything else! Worms might think that we were very important! Rats, or insects might think we were very important if we were dead, because we would then become something to eat, something to live on – but that doesn't mean to say that we are important.

It only matters, because we think we are important. That is part of the reason of why we are analysts; but the other part of why we are analysts is because we know that we are unimportant and if we don't look after ourselves and our minds, nobody else will. If we don't learn how to cure our own physical and mental defects, nobody else is going to do it. Not, unless you think, shall we say, that _God_ will do it. But, even that is a problem. Why, in that case, doesn't God start by making us perfect?

As it is, we have to perfect ourselves. I don't want to go too far into that somewhat obtuse discussion, and get away from this point about this actual patient. So it can come back to a situation in which the analyst says:

You are talking as if I were a very important person, as if, a very important person, would treat you, as if you're very important. Now, I think that would be very nearly true, if I were your mother or father and if

I had given birth to you. That might make you think that I was very important; and if I loved you like a father or mother, that might make you think that you were very important. But I'm not a blood relation, and you are in a hospital. So, why would you think that I, or anybody, wanted to bother about you, who needed a hospital?

Now, here I can talk in that way, but when you are treating the patient that's another matter, because I can say that kind of thing here, but whether it would be wise to say it to the patient is another story. So, one can come back to the point, namely: when the patient talks to you like this, what are you to say to him?

There's a difficulty which I could say a little bit more about, namely: what language are you going to talk? That depends, partly, on what language you can speak yourself; but it also depends on whether the language you talk, is the kind of language, which your patient would understand. So, quite a lot is involved in this matter. You have to know what your vocabulary is and what your language is and what language and vocabulary, your patient would understand.

T: (P3) is asking – when you refer so frequently to the words, language and vocabulary – the analyst's language and the client's vocabulary – if your meaning refers to the analyst, as someone who has an experience. I don't think she's talking about feelings of transference – but rather the experience that pours out of the analyst. And if his language is a language based on the fact that the analyst is who he is, and if you also mean – by the client's vocabulary and language – the fact that the client is what he is and expresses his being, in such and such a way.

Bion: He does, yes. In exactly the same way, as it matters what language a baby understands and speaks and what language the mother of that baby speaks and can make understandable to the child. But, that does depend on who or what the mother is and who or what the baby is.

I can make that point clearer by taking a rather exaggerated example – exaggerated but quite common – namely: there are such things as what we call battered babies. It can seem to be almost incredible that mothers and fathers can batter a newborn child.

So, you can get all sorts of people who are able to have babies, and babies can have all sorts of experiences, even before they are born! Before they are born, there can be attempts to abort them and so on… and after they are born the same thing. So, when somebody comes to you and says – apparently correctly – that they are thirty-eight, it's quite a problem as to know how they've come to exist for thirty-eight years. That's a long time.

It may not be at all surprising, that we see the patient in a hospital when you consider, where they may have been between the time when they were born and the time when they are thirty-eight. Now, part of that depends on what I call *happenings*, but partly, also, it depends on who or what the patient is, or who or what it is that has enabled them still to be in existence. So, when you see the patient, a man physically who is thirty-eight and is presumably mature – physically mature. When you say he's got a man's mind, as well character and personality, then there is a problem. The general question is: how has he come to exist? Where has he been and what has he seen, since the time he was born and now?

Now, in one sense, the general question doesn't matter to us. It's only a kind of framework, in which particular instances crop up. Now, what analysts are dealing with, is not the general principle, but the particular instance. Not the human race – because we only see one person at a time – but a *particular* person.[4] In this instance a particular character reputedly thirty-eight years old.

Now, what age is this character who thinks that the analyst is and behaves as if the analyst was a very important person and that this very important person can spend time looking at him as if he were a very important person? What age is he? The physical fact of his being thirty-eight we needn't bother with it, because it would be no good telling him that he is thirty-eight. He knows all that. So, the one question would be: what age is this person, who thinks that you are a very important person and that you, a very important person, is bothering about him, as if he were a very important person?

If you were an archeologist exploring the tombs in *"The Valley of the Kings"* in Egypt and you came across the remains of Tutankhamen, you could say: where did he come in history? But, what you are investigating is not a dead body, but a live one. We are investigating what we think is the mind or character of that creature. Now, where he and we come in history is not perhaps very important – not just at this moment – but what age he is, what age the person is, who's come to you, what <u>mental</u> age he is, *that* is important.

Again, the practical problem is: what interpretation are you to give this patient? What age are you going to interpret? That is something only you can know. You can look at one, two, three, four, five, up to thirty-eight – which do you pick? When he comes to you and talks as he has done in this session, just to use this sort of frame – that I've suggested as a kind of voluntary aid – a *Grid* in which one coordinate is: one, two, three, four, five, six, seven, eight, up to thirty-eight, or so on… where about do you place him on that 'age Grid'? Where do you place that conversation which he is having with you?

The intellectual point that we are having – that I've put to you, that doesn't really very much matter – but the practical point does. Who is talking to you? How old is he? What do you say back to him? It's a sort of archeology of the mind being done on a living object. If you were a biologist and a [strange primitive creature] was brought up in your nets, then you wouldn't have to be a simple fisherman; you'd also have to be a zoologist, to know that this specimen was a survival of a very primitive creature.

But, the same applies to us as psychoanalysts. This is what we bring up in our nets. You have caught a mind in your net. Now, as you examine it, psychoanalytically, what do you find? From what age has it survived? In what language are you going to talk to it? You must talk the language that he could be able to understand. So part of it, is you and what you've learnt – part of it – but the other part of it is what can he understand? What would he be likely to hear?

T: He suggests (P4) that the language would be what one calls interpretations, because this is an extinct language for the patient.

Bion: Yes, that will be called psychoanalysis. But the trouble is: we have to invent the language in which to interpret. What we have to interpret is what we have already seen and heard and observed in the office. So, we have to translate that into a language which the patient would be able to understand.

P4: So the vestiges of language, that the patient can understand, are understood by the psychoanalyst, who then refers to them?

Bion: Unfortunately that usually isn't the case. Unfortunately the analyst very often talks the language, which is known to psychoanalysts and psychiatrists and unfortunately patients think that they know that language, but they don't. Today, so many people think they understand psychoanalysis, because they've learnt the words, so the patient can say he's knowledgeable. Or, they often use psychiatric terms. You'll sometimes get a patient, who says that he thinks that he is _schizophrenic_, or that he thinks that he is _paranoid_. They don't know what paranoid means – those are technical terms. We may know, but we've had many years of training, medical training, psychoanalytic training. So, it's very easy for us to get taken in by a patient who talks about feeling paranoiac, but he doesn't know anything about _paranoia_ – even psychiatrists have got a lot to earn about it. So, the problem there is not to be taken in by the apparent knowledge.

This man of thirty-eight can act exactly like a man of thirty-eight and we can get taken in by that, too. So, we get back to the point: is this thing, which is occupying a body of thirty-eight and is able to act as if he were a man of thirty-eight, what age is it? What is a man of thirty-eight, with a mind of thirty-eight what he's wanting to tell you, or pretending he is, or acting as if he were thirty-eight doing in a hospital? Is he a psychiatrist? Is he a doctor? If he is, then, why is he a patient? If he says he's a patient, why does he want to be treated as if he was a psychiatrist or psychoanalyst, or a man of thirty-eight?

Now we can't say any of that to the patient, because if we did the patient would think we were being extremely hostile. So, you get up again to this fact: the practice of psychoanalysis is very difficult – it doesn't matter who it is, how experienced – it's much easier for me *to talk about* this here, than it would be for me to see that patient. So, don't be surprised to find that it's very difficult being a psychoanalyst. It's much easier *to talk like* a psychoanalyst;, much easier to read and talk like a psychoanalyst: much more difficult for me *to be* an analyst.

If you were unkind you could say to me: *"We'll stop talking about it, I'll send you the patient"*. So, I'm not really trying to minimize the difficulties, which I know you have, nor do I want to magnify them – because I know they are bad enough, anyway. That's why I think it is worth discussing these matters here – not because any of us *can tell you* what to do – but between us we might get an idea or two. I hope sometime or another, we'll even discuss this problem of the language, which we need to talk *before* it has become polluted, devalued, depreciated.

Here again we've got to stop.

Notes

1 Editor's Note: In this supervision and the supervisions that follow, A refers to the presenting analyst, T refers to the in-person translator who was assisting during the supervision, P1, P2, etc. refers to comments made by a participant in the audience during the supervision.

2 Editor's Note: The original transcription refers to this patient having been discussed previously in Supervision A17.

3 Editors' Note: It seems the participant is asking if perhaps the patient's curiosity and concern about the analyst's private life is connected to a change in the analyst produced by the earlier supervisory presentation and discussion.

4 Editors' Note: In the original transcript, Junqueira has added: I think this statement made by Bion is of fundamental importance for the technique of psychoanalysis. For example, we are used to speaking about Oedipus Complex, as if it had a practical meaning in analysis. It does not, since every one has, like fingerprints, his\her own Oedipus Complex.

Supervision A13 commentary

Marli Claudete Braga

While preparing my comments about Supervision A13 (held in São Paulo in 1978), I was overtaken by growing interest. Led by curiosity and enthusiasm, I sought in other supervisions by Bion references to the topics addressed here. While doing that, I formed an overview of Bion's working method in these supervisions, becoming more interested in general ideas, rather than dwelling only on the specific instance. Thus, although I will use Supervision A13 as an axis, I will interweave themes that stood out for me with references to these topics in other contributions by Bion.

In a general overview, I observed some of Bion's comments, such as his mentioning in one of the supervisions that his preferred vertex is that of broadening the contact of the analyst with the experience that he is living in the supervision, rather than the analyst's approach to the practice of analysis. Bion develops his work in close contact with those who are present in the supervision; he focuses his attention primarily on what is occurring at the moment. For example, in several supervisions, Bion asks the presenter if he minds being interrupted at any moment. The presenter says he does not mind being interrupted, and Bion tells the participants that they can also make observations or comments, adding that this is meant to make better use of the time. He insists on these comments in different supervisions. He also proposes (Supervisions A48 and A49, for example, held in São Paulo in 1978) that if the participants want to make any question, observation, or comment, that they should not be worried and should speak what they think and make suggestions, whatever they are. He also questions about the impressions of each one of them and if they have something that is mobilizing them. He questions: *"Any other things that strike you about it?"(...)... "Is anybody else here feeling touched?" (...)... "but, do you feel touched by this story?"* (Supervision A50, São Paulo, 1978). *"...what noises do you hear now?" "Now, where do you think you get the best view? It doesn't matter where I get it from. You can choose where you would stand, to understand what this patient is talking about"* (Supervision A37, São Paulo, 1978). He complements that by saying: *"...the advantage of a discussion of this sort is: to explore your own impressions and your own feelings about what the story, as you hear it, or as you would formulate it yourself, your version of it"* (...) (Supervision S10, Brasília, 1975).

DOI: 10.4324/9781003439233-3

In some supervisions, Bion even asks those who are present to write down on a piece of paper the first impressions that they had about what they had heard, asking them to write any idea – any one – and enumerate the order in which they wrote them, then fold the paper so as not to look at it anymore, suggesting that they hide it from themselves so that they do not know what they wrote. And he explains: *"...what I said before in terms of not keeping to memory or desire. Memory: the past; desire: anticipation. So, by hiding what you've written, it is like forgetting it"* (Supervision A1, São Paulo, 1978).

With this done, he opens the field for conjectures, removing the illusion that the analyst, those who are listening, and even himself (Bion) know, in fact, about the patient. He places himself in the same conditions as the participants and, in some moments, after listening to those who are present, he speaks about the effect created on him and about his questions and comments.

He points out that to speak about the patient is fallacious and that the supervision is meant for us to learn how people think, and not to talk about the patient; to know what we think beyond what is already there.

He continues: *"We can take advantage of this situation, both: to get an idea how somebody else does an analysis and also to consider how we would do it, if we were the analyst"* (Supervision A40, São Paulo, 1978).

I reflect: when we look over the way that Bion conducts the supervisions, I believe that we are confronting the practice of his theory of psychoanalytic observation, stimulating in us the development of this condition, proposing to us to detach ourselves from preconceived ideas, which includes the theories that underpin the psychoanalytic method.

The important thing is the experience that each one actually has about what is created in the analytical relationship, what is observed and what is possible to develop in the contact. Bion proposes that the work of the analyst is to be in contact with what is happening at the moment in which it happens: the pain that is being experienced and the shape that it is taking. He emphasizes the emotional experiences, the capture of thoughts without a thinker, instead of ready-made explanations stemming from theories. Thus, the focus no longer falls on the content, on the factual: it changes the vertex of the analytical work, which ceases to be a therapeutic method geared toward the treatment of psychopathological events, understood by explanations based on mental dynamics that psychoanalysis itself has already developed (theories of mental development and personality functioning). We could say that Bion's general idea is to move beyond the linearity of cause-effect relationships, and he cautions that if we stick to sensory data, we will be involved in an imitation of psychoanalysis.

With this, Bion removes the emphasis on the interpretation of *meanings* of mental content and favors the *meaning* of the elements that emerge in the analytical field. Thus, we propose to come to grips with two issues: the concern to develop a scientific method of observation and the attention to communication in psychoanalysis. And all these things are not to be known beforehand, but to be emergent and experienced in the intimate contact between two individuals in the analytical room.

Specifically about Supervision A13, I select below three thoughts elaborated by Bion on this supervision.

1. What is important is the patient; we are not important

Bion speaks right at the beginning of this supervision, making several observations, unlike some other supervisions in which he first wanted to listen to those who were present. He seems to have been already captured by something in the first communications, something with no association with the meaning of the words spoken by the presenter.

In regard to the description of the patient interpreting the delay of the analyst as a change in the analyst's methods, Bion offers a long comment about the psychoanalytic reasons for the analyst to treat with much discretion his personal life.

He initially mentions the importance of the analyst not telling the patient about his private life, his difficulties, because this would stimulate ideas in the patient, which may not be in any way important. He mentions:

> *Now, if I don't tell the patient anything about my private life, it's not because I've got anything to hide particularly. I don't really mind very much, but I don't tell anything because it leaves them more space in which to use their imagination.*
> (Supervision A13, São Paulo, 1978)

After several considerations, Bion seems to have reached a limit and says: *"I don't want to go too far into that somewhat obtuse discussion, and get away from this point about this actual patient"* (Supervision A13, São Paulo, 1978). However, he himself resumes this discussion and talks a little more about these ideas.

I think that Bion tells us here, in practical terms, what he told us in *Attention and Interpretation* in a more theoretical form:

> *This information is worthless at best and, at worst, harmful because every analysis is unique; talk about analysis is not.*
> *The analysis must focus his attention on O, the unknown and unknowable. The success of psycho-analysis depends on the maintenance of a psycho-analytic point of view; the point of view is the psycho-analytic vertex; the psycho-analytic vertex is O....*
> (Bion 1970, p. 27)

Continuing the approach to this topic, Bion argues that in fact we, analysts, are not important people. What is important in the analytic consultation is what the patient thinks. He insists: we are just ordinary people. The only things that are important in the analysis are the thoughts of the patient, the ideas of the patient, the feelings of the patient. He mentions that we would be important if we were the patient's mother or father, if we had given birth to him. However, he ponders: *"...here, I can talk in that way, but when you are treating the patient that's another matter"* (Supervision A13, São Paulo, 1978).

2. The issue of the language in psychoanalysis

This is a topic to which Bion returns in his interventions in this supervision, as well as in several other supervisions and writings. He systematically emphasizes the great difficulty of putting into words one's lived experience and transmitting it. There is the speech of the patient and that of the analyst, the latter being just one more occurrence: it is only one of these events. There are two individuals in the analytical room who do not know what to talk about with one another. Is it possible to talk in another way? It depends on whether the language that you speak is the type of language that the patient would understand. Thus, there is a lot involved in this issue.

> *You must talk the language that he could be able to understand, so part of it, is you and what you've learned – part of it – but the other part of it, what can he understand? What would he be likely to hear?*
>
> (Supervision A13, São Paulo, 1978)

It is essential to speak the language that he (the patient) is able to understand and that he (the patient) would be able to listen to. *"... We have to invent the language in which to interpret (...) unfortunately patients think that they know that language, but they don't"* (Supervision A13, São Paulo 1978). Bion says that it is important not to be led by the appearance of knowledge and by the difficulty of giving the interpretation. He speaks of being careful of what we say and doing so in a way that the patient doesn't feel that we are hostile to him. He also discusses the intonation of our voice. In another supervision (Supervision A49, São Paulo, 1978), he gives an example: *"... analysis itself is like songs without words, or words without songs."* How can one take care of the musicality in one's voice?

Language is not limited to spoken words; nonverbal communication is also present. Bion questions: *"...as to why, as analysts, we think verbal communication is a way of dealing with the problem"* (Supervision A33, São Paulo, 1978).

He mentions:

> *Now, as a matter of fact, the kind of thinking and the kind of talking that we do in analysis is not ordinary talking, it's not even about an ordinary subject; so, it can be very difficult for the patient to know that she doesn't know much about psychoanalysis or, for that matter, about thinking.*
>
> (Supervision A49, São Paulo, 1978)

And he says: what the patient is formulating has to do with the relationship with the analyst; with the intersection between them both; with the possible meeting place between the two. There is always an experience happening in the analytical room; if we do not perceive it, something is wrong.

I will now synthesize my overview of these formulations. I notice the extent of the analytical task when I share with someone his/her emotional pain while seeking to shelter them, to transform the experience and find a language that gives an idea about the depths of the soul, as well as the emotional bond that is being experienced between us. Some difficulties strike me: how to tune in to the experiences, to the emotional pain that is transmitted verbally to me and not even perceived by the patient? How to approach what is indeed essential using words? What 'language' does the patient speak? And in what 'language' can I speak so he can hear me? And, also, in what 'language' can I express my experience? Bion, no longer concerned with explanations or increased knowledge, but with the quality of the communication, suggests for us not to use a sophisticated or damaged (jargon) language, but one that is precise and helpful in creating thoughts. He says: *"...we'll even discuss this problem of the language, which we need to talk before it has become polluted, devalued, depreciated"* (Supervision A13, São Paulo, 1978).

3. The difficulties of being a psychoanalyst

I have selected some considerations by Bion in this or other supervisions, referring to the difficulties of *what it is to be a psychoanalyst*. I think they are important stimuli to think about our work. Nothing is more useful than to perceive these observations as posed by Bion himself, as we can read in his supervisions.

Starting with clinical practice, he tells us it is: *"... much easier to read and talk like psychoanalyst: much more difficult for me to be an analyst (...)"*. And he specifies, *"... now, what analysts are dealing with, is not the general principle, but the particular instance"* (Supervision A13, São Paulo 1978). Three years before, in Brasilia (1975 Supervision S10), Bion told us *"... practice of analysis seems to me to be an extremely difficult occupation and which hardly, hardly provides space for a dogmatic statement."*

In *Transformations* (p. 46), Bion says: *"The psycho-analyst's domain is that which lies between the point where a man receives sense impressions and the point where he gives expression to the transformation that has taken place."*

In another supervision (Supervision A37, São Paulo, 1978), Bion discriminates the difference between the theoretical study and the condition proper to the analyst, emphasizing the importance of the latter:

> *You don't have to read books by Freud or Melanie Klein and so on, only; that's quite useful – but you can read the story of your own life. For example: are you able to remember some period of your life, when you could feel like this, or understand what the patient was saying?*

In Supervision A32 (São Paulo, 1978), he adds, *"...but, you also have to read the book that is open before you, when the analysand comes into your office."*

Bion speaks to us about the challenges of giving interpretations:

If you had been doing analysis as long as I had, you shouldn't bother about an inadequate interpretation. I have never given any other kind!! That seems to me to be the real life and not psychoanalytic fiction. The belief in the existence of a psychoanalyst, who gives correct and adequate interpretation, that seems to be part of the mythology of psychoanalysis. (...) See, what I said doesn't matter; what does matter is what was going on before the eyes, ears and senses of the analyst.

(Supervision S10, Brasília, 1975)

Bion includes in this experience of the analyst and the patient the pictorial images that emerge, the 'dreaming' of what is said in the session. His conclusion is emphatic: all these things will make the practice of psychoanalysis very difficult.

So I'm not really trying to minimize the difficulties, which I know you have, nor do I want to magnify then – because I know they are bad enough, anyway. That's why I think it is worth discussing these matters here – not because any of us can tell you what to do – but between us we might get an idea or two.

(Supervision A13)

It occurs to me that in these supervisions, most of which date one year before his death, we are being greatly favored by receiving a lively 'concentrate' of decades of elaborations about his psychoanalytic knowledge. For example, he no longer emphasizes learning from experience; he rather emphasizes the emanations of reality and the importance of putting himself (the analyst) in union with this. He also proposes being available to the infinite; his basic reference is no longer the unconscious to the conscious, but rather, the finite to the infinite. Another important point is the withdrawal of an emphasis on the theoretical knowledge of the analyst, which leads the patient and his thoughts and feelings to the central position of the analytical work. With this, he proposes to the analyst to choose his own vertex, which will require him to tolerate his helplessness and loneliness.

I would like to end these reflections with a personal observation: to be a psychoanalyst is to be able to be oneself and develop one's own possibilities, and not only to learn about who one is.

References

Bion, W.R. (1970). *Attention and interpretation.* London: Karnac, 1984.

Bion, W.R. (1965). *Transformations.* London: Karnac, 1984.

Bion, W.R. (1975). Supervision S10, held in Brasília. Audiotape transcription by José Américo Junqueira de Mattos.

Bion, W.R. (1978). Supervisions A1, A12, A13, A32, A33, A37, A40, A48, A49, and A50, held in São Paulo. Audiotape transcription by José Américo Junqueira de Mattos.

Chapter 2

Supervision A12

A: I have the impression that the patient is tormented, worried… The session starts with his complaint that it is futile, that it is useless to undergo analysis, because he cannot be married. He likes his lover – his sweetheart – and he is afraid of getting married, because of his great fear of being homosexual.

Bion: Can we stop at that point at the moment? Has everybody understood?

T: It seems that everybody understands English except him, so I'm just…

Bion: Oh, I see. Has anybody… would anybody like to volunteer what their impression is, that they have so far? Suppose you were the analyst and had that experience. It's no good going on with the analysis when we heard that from the patient, do you agree?

P1: [Why has he come?]¹

T: if it's [analysis that is] not worthwhile, why does the patient come? Did he give a reason?

P1: But still he's there, he's coming.

Bion: Does anybody like to make any further suggestion about that?

P2: I feel that maybe it's useless for him I don't know… I felt that Dr. X saw him as dramatic and that maybe it's useless to help him, with this kind of problem.

Bion: Suppose this patient gets the idea that it's worth coming again, on _this_ day, so much that, he actually comes. That raises your point: why has he come? Why has he put his voluntary muscle into operation, to bring him into the consulting room? We don't have to ignore what we have already been told by the patient, namely: that the analysis is useless – we can agree with that, but then, why has he come? Now, could it be that there's some truth in the psychoanalytic theory of transference? Is it possible that the patient feels that the analyst is an attractive and comprehending mate? At the same time he's aware that the analyst's a man. So, it's no good, it can't lead to a marriage. It's no good going on with his courtship, this relationship in which he can be understood, listened to, talked to, but they're never going to marry! So, what's the use?

DOI: 10.4324/9781003439233-4

Anyway, suppose it's something like that. That's very theoretical, it's very psychoanalytical. But, this is a practical analysis, it's not a theoretical discussion of a psychoanalytic theory. So, what is the analyst to do? What would you or I say, or do, in reply to the patient's statement? Should we agree: *"Yes, it's no good! So, you don't need to come again, you've finished?"*. I don't think so, because the patient has come again this time, therefore it would be useful at any rate, according to analytic theory, to give the patient an interpretation. That's alright in theory, but what are we to do in practice? What are we to say to this patient? Well, I've interrupted this story very early so to give us a chance to discuss it. But, shall we listen to what the analyst <u>did</u> say or do? Shall we go on with the story? But first of all: I'd like to suggest that we, all of us, think what we should do… commit ourselves to this rash statement before we hear what the analyst did do. Go on!

A: Now, I think I am contaminated by the patient and I feel blocked to go on, because I'm afraid that I would tell stories about the patient.

Bion: The analysand would be contaminated too if you didn't say anything, by your silence; and he'd be contaminated if you said anything. So, I don't think there's anyway of giving the right interpretation. In another four or five hundred years, perhaps, people will give correct interpretations, but not us. We are at the birth of psychoanalysis, and it's only been going for a hundred years or so and that isn't much!

A: I think that I told the patient: *"you describe this as a sensation. I think you try to show me that you refer to something not mental, something physical, in your body"* and the patient said: *"I know this, but what should I do with this?"*

Bion: It's quite an important question. Many people feel what is the use of knowledge anyway? So, if he knows already, there's no use. What is an analyst to tell a patient, who already knows all the answers? You'll often get a patient who either goes on talking as if they hadn't heard what you'd said or else, whatever the analyst says: *"yes, I know. Yes, I know"*. They brush aside the interpretation, because they know all the answers. So, there's no room to learn anything. That doesn't mean to say that the analyst is wrong. It's quite a difficult problem what to say next when the patient says: *"yes I know"*; actually, it's very much the same when the patient says: *"I don't know what you're talking about"*, it's tempting to reply: *"I know you don't"* or *"since you know everything, it's no good going on with it"*. But, I think that one has to resist that temptation, and nevertheless, persist with whatever things one can say or do. But, I do want to suggest that I would regard that statement as being one of these fundamental remarks the: *"yes, I know"* type of intervention. It gets worse, because there are so many people who wouldn't dream of having an analysis, but they think they know all about it. So, they really do believe that the analyst hasn't got anything to tell them.

Well, could you go on ...

A: The patient goes on remarking that now he is feeling he can't get it!, that it is very disturbing. He feels like his anus and rectum would be open and he is waiting for the entering of something – a penis for instance.

Bion: Did the patient say this?

A: Yes.

Bion: Yes, now what do you think about that?

[At this point the translator asks a question in Portuguese] *"Are they a man and a woman? because I'm translating and I lost the..."*

A: Yes, they are married.

T: He's (P1) asking a question, when he (A) referred in his interpretation about a physical sensation; where did he take this information from? From his previous experiences?

Bion: Does it matter very much? Because in the consulting room you have a chance of forming your own opinion as to where he got that information from.

T: He (P1) thinks it's important for him to know, because after that, a whole train of information came on the same line.

Bion: Yes, but what strikes me about it is; I'm quite prepared to believe he has this irritation in his penis and that orifice is wide open. After all, the patient ought to know – I have a particular reason to believe he's trying to tell me lies, although he may not be. But, what I wonder is: what's happened to all the other orifices? What about the other end of the alimentary canal? What about the mouth? What about the ears? Are they shut to interpretations? Why only that orifice?

Well, perhaps we shall find out, if the patient says some more. But notice: the patient is still in the room, why is he going on with this conversation, which is so useless? He's already said it, it can't get anywhere. Then, what's he doing, what's he talking about? So to start with, your statement remains valid: why is he there? He is there: it's a fact; it's a bodily physical fact, which is contradicting and is contradicted by his statement that the analysis is useless. So one wonders is there a conflict between his... well, what we call his body and his mind? Or is there a conflict between his body and his body? His anus and his mouth? Or the... digestive orifice and the auditory apparatus? Now, these are simply speculations. So perhaps again, if we could listen to some more that the patient says.

T: He wonders if he (P2) can add something now.

Bion: Yes!

T: He is questioning the fact that the patient, although he is there as a fact: bodily present and also says in his words, that analysis is useless; if he is not there, bodily present, because it's necessary that he...

P2:   Conveys to the analyst that the analysis is useful.

P3   Useful?

P1:   Isn't Useless.

T: Useless!

Bion: But, there are so many methods of communication why doesn't he use
          them? Why does he choose to be present and to make a verbal commu-
          nication? I quite agree with you that he can come for that purpose, but
          why choose that particular means of communication? I feel that, what I'm
          drawing attention to more and more and more questions and no answers.
          However, as I say, perhaps we'll hear some more, which may give a clue.

A: The patient proceeds: *"I only get rid of this anal itching when I pass gas"*.

Bion: When?

A: *"When I pass gas, gas! I think that I should pass gas without stop, to be re-
          lieved, to get rid of the woman that I feel inside me"*. I asked him: *"Which
          woman?"* he replies: *"I don't know, if I could know"*.

Bion: Does anybody feel enlightened? Does anybody feel disposed to give any
          interpretation?

P1:   I think I would like to know what kind of gases?

T: Gas or guesses?

A: Gas. No, no, gas.

P1:   Arh… no! I didn't understand. Sorry!
          [Lot's of laughter]

A: Intestinal gas.

P1:   Yes, I didn't understand.

Bion: In the office, the fact that a conversation is taking place, is liable to obscure
          the fact that one
          [at this point we can hear Dr. Bion letting out his breath with force]
          one's breath. So, one is evacuating gas at this end and not the other end
          of the alimentary canal. That is the worst of being the analyst, because one
          can hear the patient talking and one can hear oneself talking. So, we don't
          really notice the fact that we are
          [again Dr. Bion lets out his breath with force]
          evacuating our breath, our gas. Conversely the patient knows about
          evacuating the gas, he knows that he and the analyst are evacuating, but he
          doesn't understand that they are talking. So, it's a conversation, where the
          analyst is liable to be impressed by what the patient is saying – that it can
          hide what the patient is doing in the way of evacuating his gas. As I say,
          conversely the analysand knows he's evacuating gas, but he doesn't really
          hear the conversation.

          Now, I would find it very easy if my eyes didn't tell me that there were
          two grown men in the room. But if there were a mother and a baby in the
          room then I could understand that, perhaps, the baby was suffering from
          wind – passing gas. If the baby could only talk, the baby might be able to
          tell me that I was passing gas. Now this is a very peculiar situation: the
          situation in which they are in – as our senses tell us, as our common senses
          tell us – that there are two grow men in this room.

          So, what's happening? Well, we know that we can simplify all this by
          saying: *"Oh! well that's psychoanalysis"*. Now, psychoanalysis is a word,

which has no meaning at all. It's meaningless! But it's useful for talking about this peculiar kind of conversation. So, we'll continue to use it, we'll continue to talk about psychoanalysis, use the word psychoanalysis to refer to what we're talking about. But what are we talking about? What is the real thing? Why is it that the grown man should know about trying to get rid of the idea of this un-wanted woman by

[Dr. Bion breaths out again]

evacuating it and why does the analyst give psychoanalytic interpretations? It's a very odd situation, indeed, most peculiar! It's most peculiar that the patient is talking about something so extraordinary and the analyst is doing the same thing.

These are problems which, as analyst, we may, in time, know more about – I don't think anybody else will. I think only people like us, are likely to answer any of these questions. I haven't met anybody so far – and I've met quite a lot of people – who would be more likely to know the answers to these questions, or to find them out, than us. That's one reason why I think that it's worth sticking to psychoanalysis, that's one reason why I think that it's useful, if this analyst will go on making himself available to this patient who tells him how useless psychoanalysis is.

As a matter of fact, we all know how useless analysis is; it's brought home to us everyday of our lives. We are so close to psychoanalysis, since we are psychoanalysts, that we know its faults, its weaknesses, its impotence, it's effectualness, only too clearly. What is so difficult is to know whether it works at all and if so, why? If we knew that, then we'd know why this patient had come again, why the patient was going on, trying to give the analyst information, when he's already said that it is useless, when we ourselves have every reason to know about the weaknesses of psychoanalysis.

None of the opponents of analysis can tell us as much about the defects of analysis as, those we already know. So, the patient even thinks he's telling the analyst something he doesn't know, but what he doesn't know is what is some use about it. To change into a rather different subject, in a way the child doesn't know why she has to learn the alphabet, the child doesn't know why it has to practice the piano, play, say the piano, or play with a violin, or a clarinet, or a flute and so on… but if he'll stick to it long enough, he may find out – one day he may know what music is and how to make it. In the meantime, he has to learn it when he doesn't know. So, does this patient – only it isn't the piano, it isn't spelling and he won't know coming for analysis what is the use for it, unless he has some. Then, he may discover that he's quite right: he'll never marry his analyst and his analyst will never marry him. They will never have sexual intercourse, he'll never have a breast or a penis put either into his anus or into his mouth and it would be no good putting it into his ears, anyway. So he doesn't know why he should have these sounds put into his ears, or why he should keep his ears open – but perhaps he'll find out.

Perhaps, if the analyst will go on analyzing him, the patient will find out what the use of analysis is – as a matter of fact, so will the analyst; it takes an awfully long time before one really believes that there is such a thing as mental pain and that these peculiar conversations really work. So that, one could say to Macbeth: "yes, in four or five hundred years we shall minister to a mind diseased". Today, we ourselves will discover that we can help – it actually helps to be able to have the kind of conversation, which we've been hearing something about. It's quite a surprise; it's quite a surprise, to discover that patients – this particular patient – actually improve. In fact I think, hearing it as second hand that this patient is improving.

While he is telling us of the uselessness of analysis, he is not noticing that he is improving. But if he goes on long enough, he'll notice that he's better. Sometimes, you can get situations, in which, you feel really one might just as well be talking to a wall as talking to a patient and then; by accident, you hear somebody say how this patient has improved. So, while the analyst and analysand don't know anything about it, somebody may notice that he is improving! Mind you, this does not exclude the fact that there are plenty of people who are quite capable of using analysis in order to be able to go on going down hill. I don't know if you have the expression of what is called "a loser" – a person who loses, always loses, he's always on the losing side!

Bion: And such a person can very well use analysis to the same purpose, of losing more and more. A loser can sometimes hate the analyst because he's better! He may even say: "Of course I'm better doctor, but it's nothing to do with this". So, I think that one has to get tough and pressure on. People will say: "well, of course the patient would never do anything wrong with them and they'd get well, anyway". I don't think it's true, at all.

We've again come to the end, haven't we?

A: Thank you very much.

Bion: Well, thank you very much. I've seemed to have been taking up so much time talking!

A: Yes, I think it was very illuminating for me.

Bion: Well, I think it is helpful to discuss this kind of thing, because the analytic job is so lonely! The analyst is – as it's brought home to him all the time that he's all alone. Your best source of information, help, assistance, is the patient. So, if there's anything… anyway in which, the patient can help and cooperate, it's the best help that the analyst will ever get. But sometimes it's nice to be able to exchange views with some of our colleagues.

A: Quite!

Note

1   Editors' Note: From the tape, one gathers that P1 has a poor command of English and what he wanted to say was: "Why has he come? Why did he come?"

Supervision A12 commentary[1]

Gisèle de Mattos Brito

I often say that Supervisions conducted by Bion make up a theoretical-technical treasure in which we have the opportunity to watch the author develop his thinking and conjecture on what he experiences with the impact of the clinical case presented and the attending group. In this particular Supervision, we can follow Bion on some issues that are very dear to him and that can be identified in several of his writings and supervisions.

The first point I will raise and which I think is the most significant one and the reason for our work is: Bion shows us how much he feels that psychoanalysis is a powerful and useful conversation and that, even though the patient may not know it, we must be open and available to turn his/her disconnected words into melody, into words that may make sense to the patient and the analyst together.

Bion makes us realize that he knows what he is doing – and likes what he is doing; how he sees and feels a meaning in what he does; ultimately, he shows us his deep love for psychoanalysis. He highlights the huge importance that psychoanalysis has in dealing with topics that only it is able to deal with, i.e., when a person does not know who he/she is and cannot find in him(her)self a meaning for his/her existence. Psychoanalysis enables the building of a nest to welcome, transform and label mental pain, which, in fact, exists.

Like Virgil, Bion enlightens us on the paths his sight reaches. Faced with the patient's speech that analysis is useless, futile, he inquires: *Why has he come? Is it possible that the patient feels that the analyst is an attractive and comprehending mate?* I think these questions summarize the two lines of thought that Bion developed in this supervision, the difficulties in the patient's forming a couple with the analyst and in tolerating not knowing.

Would the patient be frustrated about not being able to marry the analyst, since he is a man? As Bion rightly points out, "But they're never going to marry! So, what's the use?" In this case, would the patient be attacking the analyst for not being a partner who would meet his sexual desires? Wouldn't the analyst put his penis in the anus of the patient who hallucinates during the session? In this case, the analytical conversation would be useless, because it would not meet the concrete desire, without distinguishing among fact, fantasy, and representation, of the patient to be penetrated by the analyst.

DOI: 10.4324/9781003439233-5

The analyst is disconcerted, he finds it difficult to speak and says he fears being contaminated by the patient, to which Bion signals something very important: in the analysis room we, as well as the patient, are contaminated, either by each other's speech, or by silence; i.e., we are impacted anyway, and therefore we need to find some form of "giving correct interpretations". Nevertheless, would this be possible, even in four, five hundred years? It is likely that Bion was referring to the possibility of developing tools for greater proximity to the truth since truth itself is unknowable.

To me, it seems especially important and significant that Bion does not depart from the homosexual fantasy present in the field of analysis, and that he seems to be the only one to keep that impression in mind. He signals that he wants to hear more; that he is open to the speech of the presenter and the analyst. He does not rush into giving an interpretation, he does not saturate the field. On the contrary, much like his way of working, he inquires. One of the participants, faced with the tense atmosphere originated from the patient's speech about the fantasy of having his anus open, waiting for a penis that would penetrate it, asks: *Where did he take this information from? From his previous experiences?*

Bion asks: *Does it matter very much?* He draws attention to the fact that, in the office, we have the opportunity to directly confirm the observations of what happens in the analysis room. This is his working method, which he so well seems to take care of: to work with opacity of memory and desire, free to welcome the new, from O, so as to be open to the unknown present in each analytical meeting, open to the evolutions from O to K and from K to O.

What Bion brings us in the aftermath seems very interesting to me. He goes on to talk about his conjecture; the ambivalence he captures in the patient, and asks: How can the patient be closed through all orifices – mouth, ears – and open only through his anus? Bion raises the possibility that the patient is lying without knowing it.

Bion draws a parallel between the patient's difficulty in receiving interpretations and his acceptance of not knowing, to the closing of his ears, mouth, in such a way as to create a conflict between his body and his mind: *"Or is there a conflict between his body and his body? His anus and his mouth? Or the... digestive orifice and the auditory apparatus?"*

Bion says these are just speculations. However, they enable us to observe his degree of abstraction and depth of thought. Is there any way of learning other than from the position of not knowing? If someone refuses what evolves from experience, he/she cannot learn from it. The patient may come for analysis, be there, but if his ears are not open to the emotional, the analysis will be useless, futile. Nevertheless, the patient keeps coming. Why is he coming?

At this point of the Supervision, I think that Bion simply introduces the way he thinks it is possible for us to take advantage of the contact with the experience of the analytical relationship. By discussing psychoanalysis, a 'peculiar', powerful conversation, he leads us to experience the importance of listening to the patient. The patient thinks he knows how useless psychoanalysis is, "but what he does not know is that which is useful in psychoanalysis".

It is at this point of the Supervision that I think Bion draws a particularly important parallel with the technical attitude that guides all his work, especially from *Transformations* onwards. He says

> *To change into a rather different subject, in a way the child doesn't know why she has to learn the alphabet, the child doesn't know why it has to practice the piano, play, say the piano, or play with a violin, or a clarinet, or a flute and so on... but if he'll stick to it long enough, he may find out – one day he may know what music is and how to make it. In the meantime, he has to learn it when he doesn't know. So, does this patient – only it isn't the piano, it isn't spelling and he won't know coming for analysis what is the use for it, unless he has some.*

I think that what Bion shows us here is that the patient needs to go to the session, have open ears, accept that he does not know many things, speak, if he listens, then listen to the analyst, keep speaking, "not deviate from the analysis". Patient and analyst being attentive, observing things together, session after session. What does this entail, but placing ourselves in unison with experience? Working with the suspension of memory, desire, and understanding?

Analysis becomes a field of investigation that welcomes traces of something unknown, distressing. A preparation to be available to get in touch with something that reveals itself. It is a painful quality of giving up knowledge, the senses. Bion says

The first point is for the analyst to impose on himself a positive discipline of eschewing memory and desire. I do not mean that 'forgetting' is enough: what is required is a positive act of refraining from memory and desire.

It may be wondered what state of mind is welcome if desires and memories are not. A term that would express approximately what I need to express is 'faith'- faith that there is an ultimate reality and truth- the unknown, unknowable, 'formless infinite' (p. 31).

What remains present is trying not to organize experience. When we do this, we place ourselves in harmony with the possibility of greater contact with the unknown, with what evolves from psychic reality. O is psychic reality.

Bion emphasizes that achieving the state of receptivity to O, i.e., to the ultimate, unknown reality, involves pain and, therefore, resistance to transformations into Being, when becoming O. In *Transformations*, Bion (1965) uses the model of St. John of the Cross's three nights of darkness to talk about reaching the mental state that promotes transformation into O. The first night of darkness of the senses involves fear of ignorance. As Bion points out in his supervision, if the patient knows everything, he cannot feel ignorant and cannot be open to the unknown. The second night, that of faith, also involves obscurities, tolerance to not knowing, "because the 'faith' involved is associated with the absence of inquiry, or 'dark night' to K" (1965, p. 159), likewise, fear of ignorance. The third night is related to the end of the night and to the encounter with divinity, God himself. Fear, as Bion points out, is that 'becoming' may be indistinguishable from 'feeling like' God.

"The transformation that involves 'becoming' is felt as inseparable from becoming God, the ultimate reality, the First Cause. The 'dark night' pain is fear of 'megalomania'". Bion (1965, p. 159). These are pains and resistance to becoming O.

In the end, Bion brings us the observation that some patients use analysis to repeat and enhance their status of being losers. In this sense, we are facing resistance to development, to growth. On the one hand, to know everything, not to endure ignorance. On the other hand, not to know, or even to always lose, are forms of impediment to the creation of a bond, of "becoming one with", since, for Bion, the "unity of the human being is the pair" the couple, the bond. It ends with his precious experience: patient, best friend.

Note

1 Supervision held in São Paulo in 1978.

Reference

Bion, W.R. (1965). Transformation. In: *Seven Servants*. New York: Jason Aronson.

Chapter 3

Supervision D2

Bion:[1] … But, the real trouble is: you have to use these same words like jealousy, envy and so on… what is at issue here though is really felt to be an envy, or jealousy, which most people don't know about and which, paradoxically, is covered up by the word jealousy or envy, because, we all know this: *"Oh yes, I fell very envious of"*, so and so… such good pairs of terms, or whatever it is, but the envy or jealousy that she's talking about is a dangerous envy or jealousy, a frightening envy or jealousy. Now, that is very difficult to believe that you might know something about that. So, there's the trouble. You might talk about it and she might – as apparently she's fortunate enough to hear – believe that you really know what you're talking about, but the trouble is that so often patients say: "Oh, well, the analyst is just repeating the same old stuff, we've all heard about jealousy and envy", but we don't know what jealousy and envy really is, until we have experienced it.

A: I think it's very interesting what you are saying, because she said it the next day, when she lay down – it was the first thing she said: *"I haven't the courage to put to you this subject"* I asked: "What?" And she said: *"You know, it deserves courage, much courage"*. So I said, *"Maybe you are afraid of me in this moment. You are afraid that you have the courage, that maybe I will not have"*.

Bion: I think that she gets a certain degree of reassurance, because she really believes, for a moment or two that you know about jealousy or envy. But, then it gets covered up, because nothing particularly dreadful has happened – not since the previous day that she's seen you. So, the doubts come back again. Did you really understand what she's talking about, or did she really tell you what she was telling you about? In other words, is the language that you use, the language that she uses really speaking about the real thing, or is it covering up the real thing? So, I think that you do get this situation in which, although it's been once said, it really has to be said again and probably again and again and gradually it gets more under control.

DOI: 10.4324/9781003439233-6

A: This did not happen in this session. The point about envy happened last week, so it gave me the idea of bringing her reality to you. We are only talking about those two things: jealousy and envy. How they are together; how she uses one and the other. But, what I think is very interesting in the case is that she seems to me to be too interested in discussing the subject.

Bion: There is a further great difficulty, which concerns us all, because it is also important to show her how much she is afraid that you will be envious of her. How much her famous husband could be envious of you, if she comes to you, instead of going to him. Now, that is something which is rather difficult to put over, because if you say: *"You are afraid that your husband will be jealous or envious of your coming to such a famous analyst as me"*. Then, the patient thinks that you are talking nonsense, or thinks that you are being [arrogant or self-important] … or something. So, it is quite difficult to know how to put this point over to the patient.

A: This I feel every moment. Each word I say is a challenge and so I speak very carefully, because of it. When I feel she is missing the point, I go back all over again and I say: *"Listen, I don't think you believe in what I should like you to understand or what we two are discussing"*.

Bion: Well, it comes back to the same thing, that as analysts, we have to invent the tools we use, as we are using them. It sounds easy, because it sounds as if we just use the ordinary language. Well, so we do, but we don't mean quite the same ordinary things. That's the trouble. Because of this intensity, because of the power of the matter we're talking about, it's difficult to point out that in talking about certain things, we take these matters very seriously. That's why we think it's worth spending so much time and money over it. But patients very often don't believe that we know what they're talking about. So, you're sure to have to say it over and over again. She's sure to have to say it again, because she then believes that you can't have understood it the first time. Or if you say it again, that she doesn't understand it either.

A: But…. something I know, happened inside me, because this is the correct. I know it was something measured. I felt we were living a moment where my patient would perhaps be put in a hospital or something like that, because she couldn't eat, she couldn't sleep. She was completely involved with those things, like obsessive things. It was very difficult.

Bion: Well, the real problem is: what the price is that you'll have to pay either for being famous or for having a famous mate, a famous wife, or a famous husband, because that is something that you can't have in a vacuum. You have to have all the rest as well: the jealousy, the rivalry, the envy, the hate. That can be so frightening that you would never dare to be in such a position. So, it's opened up quite a vast subject, as a matter of fact.

A: As the… behaving I think is very difficult. She came, I'm not sure, with me last Friday, no, not Friday, last Thursday maybe, she came and she said: *"My son did this and my daughter did that and my mother…"* – I don't know what. So, instead of listening to what she really was telling me, I just made the point that I felt she was losing that courage she had told me she needed. She said: *"Yes, really I think... I don't feel like... the weekend is very close and you are not going to...[be available]. and so, I don't want to talk about it"*.

Bion: Yes. But, it is also this fear of really co-operating with you, because that is rather like taking off one's cover, like being naked as it were. It is taking the covering up off of one's character or personality itself. So, I think that the analytical experience, if she dares to co-operate, is really felt to be taking very great risks.

A: Yes, I think so, because she had one tentative attempt at suicide. Evidently, she tried to kill herself some years ago. Something like that. And then she had another tentative event, not of suicide, not of suicide itself, but she took drugs – she doesn't take drugs at all. She took drugs from a certain friend; it was marijuana. She just took it at work to a point that a doctor was called. She was very intoxicated and in my way of seeing things, it was secondarily another kind of attempt at suicide.

Bion: One of the problems here again about this suicide, which I think applies to everybody without exception, my experience of this is that patients feel: *"I'm going to frighten my analyst by threatening suicide, but, of course, I don't mean to commit suicide and I'll be saved, somebody will stop me"*. What they don't realize is: there may be nobody to stop them. Now, the analyst knows that there's nothing that can stop a patient from killing themselves, if they want to do so. But, the patient doesn't know that. So, you get this situation in which the suicidal patient says: *"But doctor, I know this was quite safe. I know that I wouldn't kill my self because I took the telephone, I called Dr. x and Dr. x came around and saw me at once"*. Can you imagine anything more ludicrously unsafe? Because, the other: the analyst, or the doctor friend, might have been in the lavatory, might have been anywhere. He might not have been there, or as a matter of fact, although she rang up, she did not succeed in talking to this person, because at that moment, she crashed, she had already taken the overdose. Now, by an extraordinary chance, this doctor suspected what happened, he came straight to this house and at once, applied the appropriate remedies and so, her life is saved! But, she never really realized that there was the slightest reason why she shouldn't take anything in excess and this is one of the problems. A patient will threaten suicide and they don't believe that it does any harm at all, except frighten the analyst and it never occurs to them that, in fact, the analyst may know that they might overstep the mark.

A: That's a very difficult point with this patient, I don't get any notice that she wants to kill herself, but I feel afraid. Sometimes she begins a sentence and I expect that she will exactly threaten me with suicide. I have it inside me, the idea that this woman is eager to kill herself.

Bion: No, this woman is eager to frighten you, but, she can't frighten herself. She can make you afraid. If you are a responsible person, or if you are a doctor, or if you are her mother, you can be made afraid of it; because, you know how dangerous it is, but the child, the patient, doesn't feel that there's any danger in this thought – it doesn't frighten her! So, she can threaten suicide and not be the slightest bit frightened. It's only the analyst who can be frightened. So, it's one of the situations in which the analyst, parent, the grown-up, the father, they are the people who can be frightened, not the child, not the irresponsible patient. Of course, the opposite of this is: to try to put this point over, in which case, *you*, then, are dangerous, because *you* are the person who has made this patient so anxious and so frightened and so forth... Well, you can't be right, not when you are dealing with somebody who is, shall we say, so infamous. There's a famous father or husband, or whatever, or brother or sister; but then, there is the patient who is equally infamous.

P1:   This word, has this word the two meanings?

Bion: Well, really, I'm trying to draw attention to the opposite of famous. There's no real language for this kind of word. We have to know something like what is meant by, say, this and then, think of its opposite; but, what language you are to use for that, I don't know. I say *infamous* but that's only making use of a very poor word for it... but if your patient's husband is so wonderful, she will be wonderful in the opposite direction. She will be a wonderfully difficult patient, or wife, or husband herself, or a famous suicide.

A: She made me very threatened by that, when she told me she was suffering very much. She said: *"I feel very anxious, very unpleasant inside of me and I feel more alive"*. Then, I was afraid when she said: *"I feel more alive"*; because, this, to me, meant like a danger that she would do something to not feel so alive.

Bion: If she is alive, she can kill herself.

A: Exactly, yes, yes!!

P2:   But, also is there a hope?

Bion: Of course, but it's so complicated! Isn't it? Because, if there's hope, then, the patient could be so jealous or envious that they'll try to kill your hope!! If I wanted to wage war against you and I thought that you hoped that you'd be able to cure me, I could do my best to make you feel that you've got a hopeless job; so that, you'd have a nasty time every fifty minutes that I saw you. If it's envy on that sort of order. So that, if there's life you can murder it, you can kill it. If there's hope you can kill the hope. So, there's a fear of any good or valuable thing, because the good or valuable thing can be killed or destroyed in some way. So, even if analysis is good, or valuable, then something can be done to get it into such a bad reputation, that nobody would ever dream of having an analysis: *"Look at the famous so and so, with the famous suicide of his wife, why? Because she went to an analyst"*. Well, it's too easy. So, I think that you are quite right about this. There's this point: you need to be cautious about these optimistic things, because while one doesn't want to be pessimistic, but one needs to be able to draw attention to both sides of it. It's like positive and negative, if you can do both of them, your point: famous, yes, but what is the opposite of famous? And so on... Hope, despair... Some of them, one can give a kind of idea of what the opposite pole of it is.

P2:   Is he not able to stand in the middle position?

Bion: Yes... well, now, this is another point. I'm reminded of, because, in fact, the mathematicians are having great difficulty over intuition in mathematics, in which, there's a denial of the excluded middle.

P2:   Excluded?

Bion: Middle. When you mention this point about somewhere in the middle, you are already raising a point that has got this huge sort of controversy even amongst the mathematicians nowadays. Whether as analyst, we can throw any light on that, I don't know. Well, we have to work this out with your practice. But, I think you are right, the immediate point is that there's nothing between these two extremes. It's all or nothing.

P1:   Can you speak about infamous? I have the feeling of infamous.

Bion: It's not that meaning I think. But, in fact, again, the ordinary language, the ordinary conversation language that we use, isn't really good enough for psychoanalysts, for psychoanalysis. So, the point that you're raising there is: what this is to be called? Suppose you want to put this over to somebody, who's not an analyst, a patient, or something like that.

P1:   It would be a moral judgment.

Bion: Possibly! You have to invent it at the time that you're doing it. While the patient is talking to you, you have to think what words you are to use, which the patient can understand. This sort of thing seems to me to be a kind of difficulty we know about, if we practice analysis. If it's just a question of reading about psychoanalysis in a book, it's really quite apparently simple in spite of these millions and millions of interpretations and theories and so on... In practice, the unfortunate analyst has to invent the language while he is listening to the patient. He's got to think of what to say; you have to explore your own mind about this intimate or new way to know what part of it to tell your analysand.

P1:   I thought of this. .... My impression of is that the patient is playing a game with the analyst, with this threat to commit suicide.

Bion: Yes.

P1:   Like playing a game?

Bion: Yes.

A: ....this moment, so difficult for the patient. I remembered something that you said, that you had introduced the patient to himself and you have to introduce the patient to himself. This *"himself"* as he is. Something like that, you said.

Bion: Yes, yes!!

A: And then, one day – those days after this break – I dedicated myself to help her to see how difficult this behavior, jealousy and envy, was; something that she had felt in the past, when her sister was born. She told me incredible things about her behavior, when the sister was born.

Bion: Yes.

A: I think this helped her a little, because she said in the end, after we discussed this: *"Well, I felt lighter"*. You know, like that. Something that she was hoping that she could feel again, lighter, and I did this for her.... and I had the idea that she was just consoling me with something she was intending to do.

Bion: Yes. That's the advantage of the actual analysis, because you've got a chance of feeling what's going on. Not simply up here,

> *[Dr. Bion probably pointed to his head]*

but somewhere inside, you can feel and that's what's so difficult about scientific meetings and such, because you are talking and one has to use a language that's all theory and it is so difficult to say to somebody: *"Yes, but I was there and I know what it felt like, because I could feel it"*. So difficult to say, especially, to people in a scientific meeting.

A: .... in a scientific meeting, anybody can just talk theory, but when you are with your patient, you feel that patient is really there, even when he is trying to tell you: *"No, I'm not"*. I think it's a difficult task really.

Bion: Yes. it would be quite useful to do just what you are saying, if you could, also, if you remind the patient that there isn't any shortage of murderous envy and hatred. Therefore, if she, or her husband, or yourself, had any danger of being famous, then you'd also be in danger of being murdered. So, there's no need of self-murder. That's a luxury, because, there are plenty of people who are perfectly willing to murder you anyway, without your own assistance. So, in some respect the suicidal impulse is, in fact, redundant. It's an unnecessary murder, because there are plenty of people who are perfectly willing to do it for you, anyway. That's the scale of this business about envy and rivalry and fame and so forth...

A: ....I tried very much to feel the atmosphere of these last sessions, very difficult, really, very threatening – my patient suffering very much.

Bion: Well, I can understand that, because, again, this is a problem of how to put over to somebody who wasn't there, what happens when you are there. This is the huge difference between the practice of analysis and the theory about it.

A: Well, in reality, this is a frustration for me, because, I would like to be able to get help from you to help me avoid my patient's killing herself... I would expect almost a miracle from you; but, anyhow, I still have the right to hope for it. So, I would like to give you more of the situation.

Bion: Yes, yes, but what is so difficult is: it's easier to believe that somebody else will be able to help. It's so hard to believe how important you are, when you are the analyst and in fact, when you are the analyst, you are all alone. The only help you've got is the analysand. Now that analysand may be able to put up with jealousy, or envy of you and help you, to help them. But the trouble is: the more your patient helps you, the more famous you become; therefore, more dangerous; the greater the jealousy, or envy of you to be so lucky as to have such a helpful analysand and so lucky as to be able to be such a good analyst. But, she doesn't know how dangerous it would be, if she chose to be a bad patient. She thinks that that would be perfectly easy as if you could afford to have a suicidal patient on your hands, in the sense of either: the patient would be prepared to kill herself, or to kill hope – to take your point – or kill off any kind of progress. This is the moment's problem: how to find a language which could explain this to the patient, in a way that the patient could understand what you're talking about and the patient would, also, know that you know what she's talking about. If she tells you of her envy, or hatred, then you would know enough to know what she is talking about and that is so difficult for the patient to believe. If she does believe it, then she gets jealous, envious; if she doesn't believe it, then she feels that she's isolated.

A: Most of the time when she finishes the session, she just stands up and goes away and says: *"Until tomorrow",* or something like that and twice she said something instead of *"Until tomorrow"*: *"Thank you".*

Bion: Right!

A: Look, everything she does, threatens me. In reality, I feel anxious the whole session. For instance, the first time she said: *"Thank you",* the first moment, I was flattered; but, today, when she went off and shut the door, really I am not flattered.

Bion: This point is quite an important point, because the patient will slip it out in words that are always *inaudible*. But, I think, if you get a chance, you can draw attention to it and say:

> *You know, two or three times recently you said 'thank you' to me. Now, this doesn't really tell me very much about what I have done, or that I've done anything, but, it does tell me a great deal about you, if you are able to say 'thank you' because that shows that you are capable of gratitude or affection.*

Now this, then, draws attention to the fact to the patient, that they have got a capacity, in spite of their jealousy, envy, or hate, or rivalry and at the same time, to feel grateful. So, if you can draw attention to that, it also makes it possible to the patient to learn that analysts aren't concerned all the time – to turn to the case that we've been discussing -with being a private detective, or finding the criminal, or something. We are also concerned with trying to draw attention to the whole of the personality, including the good or valuable things they've got. So, it's not a fault of the patient that they're capable of being grateful, or saying thank you, but, nevertheless, they need to know that they are capable of it, it even shows in analysis.

A: This is something like being able to love.

Bion: Yes, one feels that behind there must be something like that, it's just a little spurt of love. It's a little expression of it; it's a little attempt to see what happens, because, if she says *"thank you"* – to make an exaggerated story – the analyst might get furious and say: *"I don't want your thank you"*, or something like that. Well, of course, one wouldn't do anything so stupid, on the other hand, it does help if the patient feels that it is permissible, or possible, to love somebody without, as it were, being killed for loving them; even possible to love somebody who's nothing like her husband. See, loving is not a crime, it's not wicked, but it can be hated nevertheless and in fact, the capacity for love can, itself, be felt to be something which is extremely valuable. So, there can be always the fear that the love, itself, can be destroyed by the envious, or hostile person. Or, putting it in another way, that you can have a kind of analysis, in which you end up by being a person who's so theoretical, or so abstract, or so up here – Dr. Bion points to his head – that it's impossible to be loving or affectionate also. Really, for example: one could say to oneself – that's only individual – but, whether you have an analysis, or whether you don't, you may, in the course of life, became not necessarily a nicer person, because you don't become less capable of being either: lovable or loving anybody. That is the difficulty with most people in the course of life. One has such an experience of life that the capacity of love isn't so strong. So when you get a little sparkle of it – like that showing – it's a good thing to draw attention to the fact that there's a spark still alive, in spite of all the hatred, envy and so on…

A: I think the analyst, in this actual situation, feels persecuted, really.

Bion: Sorry?

A: I said, in such a situation, the analyst feels persecuted and this is no good for the patient.

Bion: It's no good for the analyst.

A: No good for the analyst!

Bion: This is one of the difficulties which are set to the analyst: all of us have to be awfully tough because we can feel.

A: Tough?

Bion: Tough, yes.

A: Yes.

Bion: Because, it is important to be able to go on being sensitive to what is going on, although the whole pressure is to become insensitive; to grow a kind of crust, so that one learns not to feel anything – It's a kind of defensive measure.

A: I just think that she has a great envy, but she has two children, she was able to have two children, then, it's something, because if you are able to have children, perhaps she would say: *"Well, I'm not so envious"*.

Bion: That is true, but there's a great difficulty; I see it in this way: personally, I am doubtful about the ordinarily accepted statement about sexuality, because I think that sexual maturity, physiological, anatomical maturity comes about very soon – I don't know when you would say it, you have to make up your own mind as to when you would say it – but, I personally would have no hesitation in saying that the person who is mature at, say, puberty, that they're a completely sexually mature person. Not, if you are an analyst; not, if you are talking about the mind, or a personality of character. Sexual love, in the narrow sense of the term, can be complete, quite complete enough to have a family and children, but not complete enough to have children after they are born, after they are growing up, after they are becoming famous. All that, you see, is really felt to involve something like passionate love – I don't know what name to give it, there's no language for it – but, it is really what we, in fact, have to deal with. We try to give our patients a chance of becoming mature characters, mature personalities. That does not occur at the same rate as what happens inside my skin; one can be anatomically and physically mature very early, but mentally no – I don't think so. Mind you, I do think that there can also be mental precocity. Say, that the patient may suffer from being too precocious mentally, for example: a girl can be extremely maternal, many, many years before there's any question of having babies, or whatever else, that's a terrible crime because, for years, she suffers the frustration, they have to wait, as it were, for the body to grow up, to catch up with the mind.

But, with most people, the body, as it were, succeeds at being married. It is as if one could say: *"Oh, yes I'm just like a married person; just like a mother, just like a mother, who has a family"*, and so on… but, that isn't the same thing as becoming one. From our point of view, what one would need to keep in mind, is that this patient of yours is just *like* the wife of her famous husband, but she isn't the wife of a famous husband. She may be becoming one, but she isn't one, not yet. Now, one doesn't say that, one keeps that to oneself, but in the course of analysis, you may have a chance to draw attention to little bits and pieces.

A: Do you think this interesting: all Brazilian wives use their wedding ring; she doesn't, she doesn't!

Bion: Does she mention this?

A: I did.

Bion: Yes.

A: I did.

Bion: She didn't. Did she know she wore it, or didn't? Did she know this? Did she know she didn't wear it?

A: Oh, yes!

Bion: She knows it.

A: She knows! It was on purpose. She said: *"I don't feel married with X why should I use a ring? It would be a lie"*. Yes, she answered me exactly that.

Bion: Yes.

A: The truth, I would say, in this case, I don't feel like questioning her.

Bion: One wonders what this ring means. See, this ring that is worn, or isn't worn. One wonders what this patient thinks this ring means, which is not, as it were, something that is valuable, or shows something that is desirable.

A: She says that it seems to her like slaves use those things, so, she won't use it.

Bion: Well, that clinches it, it's a sort of badge of inferiority.

A: Yes, dependence.

Bion: Servitude.

A: Servitude, dependence. To be a real woman of a man, is to be completely...

P1:   Chained.

A: Inferior.

Bion: What happens if you have a famous husband... I mean, is that going to be a badge of service to you, too? To have or to admit the fame of your partner; this is most characteristic, I think, of time and time again, of being a male, who seems to resent the possibility of the famous wife. That's why you get so much of this business, in which it looks as if they're married and then the woman feels that the moment you get finished with the child, bearing and so forth... there's nothing more to be said for it, because of this ridiculous business, where there can't be a famous woman, only a famous husband! Well, after all is said and done, there are women who have been famous, nobody knows how, but they do get famous. Even in my own country, I sometimes wonder how on earth there is a Margaret Thatcher, because that takes some doing. So, I think that this ring is significant and it would be useful to know what it means.

A: She said, kidding me: *"Someday I will put on my ring to be like you"*.

Bion: Yes, yes.

A: *"Never dare, I want to imagine someday I'll put it on"*.

Bion: This would be something like admitting that it was valuable or useful to come to you. It's really like saying: *"Thank you"*, and people would know about it. That she'd have to be prepared to admit that she'd come to you for analysis and that it helped her. But, this tiny spark of love which might grow up and that anyone might know about it. Of course, to go further than this, then: is loving somebody a sign of servitude? Is it a sign of inferiority, to be capable of loving somebody? Is the only way of being famous to be a sort of murderer or the mass murderer? Sometimes, one feels in a sort of male civilization, the sign of fame is to be the person who is responsible for the death of thousands. To be a sort of Hitler: the more people you can kill, the more famous you are.

A: What you said, that the body can be grown up, not the mind, that you may have a special life and still be a little girl in your mind. I wonder if it's no good to show to the patient that there is not this same movement in the mind and in the body, that they are not synchronized...

Bion: This is the problem, all this, of how you are to make this clear to the patient, because you've got to talk the language that your patient can understand. See, here we can discuss these matters, but we have much more experience than the patient has. With your patient, your problem is: how to say that to her. It sounds so simple, but, in fact, it's difficult. All that one can say about it is: you have to try talking a language, which conveys what you want it to convey, and at the same time, which she could understand. Have you got any example in mind, of where that particular problem crops up?

A: No, but, I have an association, I was speaking about another patient of mine, that the envy is also so visible and she's not able to have babies, all hers; the problem is around this problem, of not being able to have babies.

Bion: That she wants to be part...

A: She wants, but she can't and she helped a lot of children in her work.

Bion: She helps but she has to borrow somebody else's children...

A: To work with.

Bion: So that she wants to have children, but she's got to have a mother who will produce the children for her. Well, I think you have got to come to it from all sides. Take up little bits at each time, but the point about it... that you can see the picture as a whole. You can see the problem there and when a little bit of it shows up, you can interpret that little bit until the bits all come together and then it's possible to show her what the whole picture is. But, it certainly sounds as if she has to be still in the same state of mind as the little girl who may have powerful maternal feelings, but has to borrow the children from somewhere as if she were not capable of having children herself. Now, if the belief that she can't have children is strong enough, then it can actually have an effect upon her. Indeed, this is one of these situations, where the thought of the idea is so powerful that it actually brings about the state of affairs that's feared. The patient is so convinced that they can't have children, that they cannot do or be whatever you have to do or be, to be capable of having children either getting so tense, or so blocked up, that really the sperm or the penis wouldn't be able to communicate or to put a child into her.

Note

1 Editors' Note: The transcript of this Supervision seems to start in the middle of a session that is already in progress. This may be due to problems with the tape, which is no longer available.

Supervision D2 commentary

Celso Antonio Vieira de Camargo

In this supervision, Bion presents us with several essential issues of analytical practice and discusses how to establish a more truthful contact with our own psychic reality. He exposes what James Joyce called "idées mères," a concept often quoted in "A Memoir of the Future," which refers to thought-generating ideas, capable of triggering an emotional state in the recipient and generating another set of new problems and issues. Bion writes and speaks in a way so as to invite his interlocutor to fill in what he exposes with his own personal experience (Hinshelwood, 1992, p. 253).

This is the idea that arises, for example, in the concepts of alpha function, alpha and beta elements, and in the entire trilogy of "A Memoir of the Future." This idea will be a constant in this supervision: only the analyst (and his patient) can experience the analytic session. However, with our own experience of life, personal analysis, and analytical work with our patients, we can make an attempt to get closer to the clinical material.

The complexity of the human relationship is clearly apparent throughout this supervision. It is a demonstration of the difficulties we encounter in the proper use of language, of intuition as a tool for contact with life, and of how emotions, here highlighted by envy, act on our alpha function, destabilizing our capacity to perceive reality, especially psychic reality.

We are faced with a person in analysis who has some striking features: she is married to a famous husband and has to deal with her envy, perhaps exacerbated by this situation, highlighting an intense self-destructive impulse. The fear of a more truthful contact with her emotional life appears almost as a corollary from this emotional organization. Initially, Bion presents us with a common difficulty in analysis: how to communicate our impressions to someone, using language that allows the person to perceive what we are talking about, a 'language of achievement'. What vocabulary can we use to make it easier for the person in analysis to get in touch with the emotional experience that we intend to show? We know that words can be used to bring us closer to something true, or to evade what would be a more genuine, yet painful, contact with our psychical reality. After all, with words we can do whatever we want: they do not protest to us at how we are using them. And there are emotional situations, as in this case, where the pain is extremely difficult to bear.

DOI: 10.4324/9781003439233-7

This case presents us with a situation that is frequently seen in the clinic: in pointing out that the patient experiences envy, and in this case, envy with extremely destructive characteristics, the patient can hear the word, which she already 'knows,' and use this everyday knowledge to move away from a deeper emotional experience of what is being shown to her.

While living, we are constantly going through emotional experiences. We inevitably experience emotions. But emotion can also be the kind of thing that leads us to evasion: "ah, envy, I know about this, I am very envious," the patient might say, and with that, they move away from really living the explosive contact with their murderous envy. The emotional experience lived in this way is, let's say, 'theoretical,' without affective resonance, and pushes away the real possibility of learning. In other situations, the emotional experience can lead to learning about our psychical life, and therefore lead to a psychical change. This can be a 'catastrophic change,' which seems to be one of the sources of the intense fear of contact with psychic reality that we all experience, and which here also threatens to emerge.

The term 'catastrophic' may be misleading in a certain sense: change becomes catastrophic when it cannot be elaborated and transformed into a creative situation. When we experience change, we have to abandon an older way of functioning, and this arouses fear and fantasies of catastrophe. As Bion says, change is catastrophic in the sense of being accompanied by feelings of catastrophe (Bion, 1965, p. 6–9). Of course, in a personality incapable of change, the questioning of 'the establishment'[1] can actually precipitate the catastrophe, *i.e.*, highlight the extreme psychic precariousness that nevertheless already exists. When, for example, fantasies of immortality, so common in adolescence, but persisting in various ways throughout life in an attenuated manner, when these fantasies are questioned in the analysis, the anguish is intense. In the Bible, we can read: "For thou art dust, and to dust thou shall return." A phrase which in my view is an example of the 'language of achievement': quickly and succinctly, we are put in touch with our smallness before life, a phrase that puts before us the anguish of annihilation, the final step of everything that is alive. The important point is that, by changing, we destroy an older way of functioning. Fear, fantasies of catastrophe, and hatred towards analysis and psychic life inevitably appear, in both the analyst and the patient.

On the other hand, if we manage to deal with the destructiveness, recognizing and learning about the characteristics of our emotional life or its destructive, invariant configurations can lead to great development. Had Oedipus succeeded in elaborating the tremendous emotional impact of recognizing that he had killed his own father and married his mother, he would have learned a lot about his parents, about himself, and about the danger of embarking on oracular predictions without using his own discriminative capacity. This perception only appears much later, in "Oedipus at Colonus," when he responds to Creon: "Come, answer me one question, if thou canst: if one should presently attempt thy life, would'st thou, O man of justice, first inquire if the assassin was perchance thy sire, or turn upon him? (2004)."

Bion also presents an interesting observation: when we are in a relationship with someone, a world of emotions is mobilized. In this case, to be related to someone famous is inevitably accompanied by envy, jealousy, rivalry, hatred, with all occurring simultaneously. In fact, I think that if we are in a true relationship, this plethora of emotions will always appear at some point if the relationship is not idealized. In a psychoanalytic experience, in cooperating with the analyst, the overly envious patient feels they are taking a great risk, which consists of having their destructiveness mobilized. To some extent, the success of the analysis has, as a counterpart, the inevitable appearance of envy.

As mentioned by one of my patients who works in the financial area: I feel great pleasure when everyone makes money from an operation. But my pleasure is much greater when my competitors lose a lot, even if I do not get anything. A practical example in my view of extremely destructive envy.

Another issue that Bion points to is the dissociative aspects at work in this case and many others: suicide may correspond to an intention to reach out to someone (the father, the mother, the analyst) rather than actually killing oneself – but the risk that the patient is exposed to is real, although he does not realize it. It is in this respect that Bion says that the patient can frighten the analyst, but not herself: her fantasy is that she, herself, is not in danger. If the husband is famous, she will be infamous, her own way of making a big impact. That is, through the 'fame' of producing, say, infamy. For example, in analysis, making the analyst become famous for having had a famous suicide among his patients.

There is a certain interesting paradox in the situation of envy: if the work develops, the patient may feel more alive, but may want to kill that life, that hope, depending on the load of envy that she presents. How can one draw attention to the positive qualities of one's mental life, how can one enable the transformation of envy into a stimulus to achieve development, without mobilizing the excessive envy of one's own psychoanalytic work, and consequently the desire to assassinate the analyst and the analysis itself? Interrupting the analysis, for example. As Bion tells us, there is no lack of envy and murderous hatred.

I think it is useful to recall the work of Melanie Klein, when she points to envy as having a constitutional base and being initially directed towards the breast, which is felt as a representative of the instinct of life and creativity (Klein, 1974). And envy constitutes a fundamental element in disturbing the creative process.

Bion also points to the difficulties that arise when the patient experiences feelings of gratitude. In this situation, the 'thank you' that the patient addresses to the analyst when she leaves the session involves a development, related to the recognition of the capacity of the analyst, and also of herself, expressed in the capacity to feel gratitude, but which brings a difficulty, which is an increase in the envious feeling. I believe that situations of this kind show what colleagues Arnaldo Chuster, Gustavo Soares, and Renato Trachtenberg have approached through the concepts of complex field and object, and which we have here called the multi-dimensional mind, a term that seems to me very suitable for the psychic life, and which has often been used by João Carlos Braga and Julio Frochtengarten.[2] The very concept of transformations and invariance as simultaneous components of the same process puts us in the position of being faced with this enigma. There is something that changes and something that remains, simultaneously. Common sense easily accompanies the idea of change, or even that of permanence in the sensory world, but the perception that permanence (invariance) and change (transformation) are both present is an enigma. The possibility of living with the paradoxes is another theoretical tool that Bion has left us. It was already present embryonically in Freud, and was intuited genially by Melanie Klein, when she conceptualized the permanent oscillation between the positions, PS↔D.

It is interesting to note that this paradox seems to have already given way to some theories among the Pre-Socratics. Heraclitus places us before the realization that the river never runs twice through the same place (for those who enter the same rivers, new and different waters run), and Parmenides of Elea tells us that being is, non-being is not. This seems to contain the notion of something that does not change in the universe.

There remains, thus, a single path: the being is. Not being begotten, it is also imperishable; it has, with effect, an entire, unshakable, and aimless structure. It never was, nor will ever be, because it is, in the present moment, entirely complete, one, continuous.

By adding any adjective to being, I distinguish and falsify it.

The feeling of gratitude shows the functioning of the creative element within the mental life. Detecting it alongside the destructive aspect is, therefore, so fundamental. Realizing the existence of the capacity for gratitude within us enables us to establish a creative relationship with our own psychic reality.

At one point, Bion presents an element of the most fundamental importance, the solitude of the analyst (and the patient) within the analytic room, and, we would add, in life. We are alone: we can have friends, help, but what we live, we do so in solitude. And solitude, if tolerated and elaborated, may contain an element of extreme creativity. The fact that we are alone means that each one of us is unique. It is interesting to note that the analyst tells Bion that she hoped he would help her prevent the patient from killing herself – "I was almost expecting a miracle from you" – and Bion replies: "It is hard to believe how important you, the analyst, are in the analytic room, because you're the only person living in that situation, apart from the patient."

We can express this idea in another way, from another vertex: instead of thinking about being alone (which may have a somewhat derogatory sense in common language), we can speak about the couple that we are able to form between ourselves and life. It is said that Michelangelo, upon finishing the famous sculpture of Moses, struck the sculpture and said: "Parla!" I think he showed us, with this gesture, that passes through the creative area of hallucinosis; the living, vibrant relationship he had established with that work. Alone. A loving relationship with himself, with his work.

A phrase from Walter Hugo Mãe (2013) enchants me, in particular: a truly loving relationship brings a certain definition to our incompleteness. I would add: a certain momentary, unstable definition, like the psychic life itself, but that is what life allows us to have.

And how does one maintain a loving relationship with life, facing all the obstacles and frustrations that inevitably arise while living? One way is to realize that psychic life cannot be 'cured', but we can learn from it, if we have the resources. Unfortunately, this possibility is hardly recognized in depth by most of our patients.

The psychic field is complex, because it has no sensory consistency, although its consequences have, and they are very significant. It is complex because it develops over time, never stays the same, as, in fact, time itself. We can say that beyond all dimensions of reality we would have to add the dimension of deep interiority. This is where, in addition to the phenomena we have learned to identify as belonging to the unconscious, there is the interpenetration of one mind into another, as shown by the phenomenon of projective identification described by Melanie Klein, which seems to me to arise in this case.

Towards the end of the supervision, other equally stimulating ideas emerge. The difference between love and biological sexual maturity, on the one hand, and what Bion calls passionate love, which relates to a more mature quality of a relationship, closer to the depressive position and consideration of the object.

We are surprised in this passage with a way of introducing an idea in a shocking way: having children after they are born, grow up, and become famous. We say 'having children,' which is the colloquial way to express motherhood or parenthood. But the children do not belong to us, and I think that in this idea by Bion we must include the ability to allow children to acquire their own identity and authority, and to have the courage to ultimately allow them to take our place. I think this is the concept of maturity, which is not about being absent from life as we get older, but about changing roles. There is a long period when we spend a lot of our time helping our children grow, but we then have to withdraw from that function, being present only when necessary, and taking care of our own development. As Bergman mentions, on Bergman Island: "I never imagined that getting old was a full-time job," and I believe he was referring to the growth that is possible, though laborious, as one ages.

One last word on the ring issue, the wedding ring that the patient does not use. Bion uses his intuition (I think it is a good example of this) to realize that, for her, the marriage relationship is experienced as a bond of slavery, or more precisely, servitude, and that this is represented by the ring. When one begins to talk about her not feeling comfortable using the ring, on the grounds that it is not true, he proposes that what is at stake is the fantasy of inferiority. I think it is an intuitive grasp of something that is represented by the ring, which was part of that person's emotional reality, and which was not immediately visible.

One of the conceptions of intuition is that it would involve direct, immediate, and complete knowledge — even if momentary — of the experience. And the term 'immediate' here means without significant participation of our reflective capacity at first (Bergson, 2006).

This supervision is a kind of practical demonstration of how intuitive thinking works: we can see an emotional configuration emerge where envy, rivalry, hatred of reality, an outline of creativity through feelings of gratitude and satisfaction with the work done are distinguished.

Finally, I want to bring up an image of Camus, in "The Myth of Sisyphus," in which he makes an analogy between our human condition and this myth. I think it serves as a model for any development – of analysts and patients.

I leave Sisyphus at the foot of the mountain! One always finds one's burden again. But Sisyphus teaches the higher fidelity that negates the gods and raises rocks. He too concludes that all is well. This universe henceforth without a master seems to him neither sterile nor futile. Each atom of that stone, each mineral flake of that night-filled mountain, in itself, forms a world. The struggle itself toward the heights is enough to fill a man's heart. One must imagine Sisyphus happy.

(Camus, 1991)

Notes

1 Editor's Note: The author is using the word "establishment" as used by Bion (1970) in *Attention and Interpretation*.

   In recent years there has grown the use of the term Establishment; it may refer to that body of persons in the State who may be expected usually to exercise power and responsibility by virtue of their social position, wealth, and intellectual and emotional endowment. I propose to borrow this term to denote everything from the penumbra of associations generally evoked, to the predominating and ruling characteristics of an individual, and the characteristics of a ruling caste in a group.

(p. 73)

2 Editors' Note: These are all prominent Bionian Brazilian authors.

References

Bergson, H. (2006). *O Pensamento e o Movente*, p. 29, Livraria Martins Fontes Editora, tradução Bento Prado Neto.

Bion, W. (1965). *Transformations*, p. 6–9, William Heinemann Medical Books Limited, London.

Hinshelwood, R.D. (1992). *Dicionário do Pensamento Kleiniano*, p. 252–253, Editora Artes Médicas Sul Ltda.

Klein, Melanie (1974). *Inveja e Gratidão (Envy and Gratitude)*. Imago Editora.

Mãe, Walter Hugo (2013). *A máquina de fazer espanhóis*, p. 84, Editora Objectiva em associação com Cosac Naify.

The Mith of Sisyphus and Other Essays, Ed. Vintage, 1991.

The Oedipus Trilogy (Oedipus the king, Oedipus at Colonus, AntigoneSófocles), p. 101, Ed. CreateSpace Independent Publishing Plataform, 2014.

Chapter 4

Supervision D10[1]

A: This patient is forty-four years old, single and he is for seven and a half years in treatment with me.

Bion: Seven and half years...?

A: Seven and a half years.

Bion: I didn't quite catch what you said to him. What happened in the seven and a half years?

A: He is in treatment with me.

Bion: Yes, I see.

A: He was graduated abroad. He lives in a little hotel. He had previously moved several times, always in a way he used to describe to me, ... because somebody around him behaved in an unbearable way, or that, for him, it was no longer possible to tolerate the behavior of these, or that person, or these or that influence around him.

Bion: This is what he told you?

A: Yes!

Bion: Recently or...?

A: From the beginning, from the very beginning.

Bion: I see!

A: Now, he is living in this hotel for nearly three years, three or four. He is not able to work.

P1:   To what?

A: To work. He only works... in this almost eight years of treatment that... he was able to earn a very little amount of money, working as a guide for French tourists, during the Carnival - a very little amount of money! Before his coming to me, he had worked regularly. After abandoning his engagement or professional compromise... He produced in Paris a kind of film considered a very good one. Some days ago, some days previous to this session...

[A phrase is inaudible]

He introduced himself to another colleague, this man had graduated ten years later[2] and this man asked him: *"Oh, you are the X,[3] oh, I saw your film there and I would like very much to meet you and I am very interested in you. I liked very much your film"*.

DOI: 10.4324/9781003439233-8

I don't recall enough, this man received monthly the money for the institute, from a relative; from an uncle. But his brother-in-law is the responsible for the admittance.

Bion: Responsible for...?

A: For the remittance.

Bion: Yes.

A: To put in the bank. But the... who furnished the money is the uncle.

Bion: Yes.

A: His uncle. A fortnight ago, more or less a month ago, he was introduced to someone. In the first interview, this man asked him whether he could be his assistant [working] in another state, other than X [his state of residence], to produce a film... a kind of... I don't know the name in English... a documentary.

Bion: Yes!

A: About Brazil. He 'showed himself a little person' [i.e., timid and without confidence] because of the treatment. But at the second interview with the man, after being with me,[4] he answered the man that he had resolved his main problem in X [his home state] and would be able to accept the conditions. When the producer responsible for the T.V. [the television producer of the project?] asked him about how much he wished to earn, he asked him: *"How much earns an assistant?"*. In this base, he was more or less conjecturing, depending upon a letter that the man, who went back to X..., who would write to him. When I came from X,[5] I didn't know the result of the situation and I am here more than one week. I have some topics, this is one session that... I don't know what...

Bion: So you're not seeing him just now?

A: Yes.

Bion: The analysis is what? Stopped or...?

A: No, only we interrupted with... because of my...

Bion: Change over.

A: Change over! Yes.

Bion: What is the idea then, is he coming again, or...?

A: Yes, we agreed that if he is able to accept the work, he would come back to proceed the treatment.

Bion: Is he going to let you know this?

A: No, I think that, don't know the word... I act in this way: he would accept the work, the project would last for sixteen weeks, then he would return.

Bion: He said this?

A: I myself - without payment.

Bion: Without?

A: Without payment.

Bion: Um hum.

A: A kind of interruption of the treatment without payment.

Bion: Yes.

A: The patient said:[6] *"Yesterday evening, I became very angry at that guest"*
- one guest they had in the hotel –
   Having he (the guest) been called to the telephone, he asked me from the counter where the telephone was - he asked me to low down the volume of the T.V. apparatus, because of the noise. He was talking on the telephone, asking me to low down - yes! Because I was seated relatively near the T.V.

Bion: Yes.

A: *"I replied to him, to ask the manager to do this, because ... when the guest finished the conversation, he approached to me, he told me not to talk to him anymore, that I was a very problematic person, (he had spoke to my patient) not work for anything".*
   He went up to his room and said: *"I didn't tell him any word and re-mained silent".* I replied for the patient: *"You have satisfied the guest's solicitation".*

Bion: Of...? Of...?

A: The guest's solicitation - the request of the guest: not to talk. The patient went on: *"I decidedly do not like that Portuguese owner of the hotel. When I entered the lobby of the hotel and spoke to him friendly his answer to me was that life was that way".*

Bion: When he complained of the other guest?

A: No, the owner of the hotel.[7]

Bion: Um hum.

A: Following my remark, it suddenly came to my mind, that he was referring to his mother - the patient's mother lives in another state, a little, more or less old... I talked to the patient:[8] *"You mean that the owner of the hotel is acquainted with your mother?"*

Bion: Can we shut the window a bit? It's a bit noisy. Do you mind if we have the window shut a bit? Everybody agreeable to that? It's a bit difficult to hear.
   [A background noise of a window being shut]

A: The other guest came back from his room to the lobby and told the patient: *"It would have been perfectly possible for you to have stretched our hand in the direction and to... to..."*

Bion: Turn off!

A: *"...to turn off the T.V.".* Then he walked in the direction of the counter, where he bought some envelopes to mail - some advertisements of his mer-chandise. I started to think that he had... that he knew... that he had the knowledge that I was a Jew.

Bion: Your patient is a Jew? Um hum.

A: *"Because he was buying the same envelopes I used to buy, though I usually buy smaller ones, to put, send my movie scripts"* - he writes movies scripts - this led me to think about Durex tape and of circumcision.[9]

   This guest is really unbearable to me, he is the one that is constantly asking me for a cigarette, for matches, all the time. He usually, he keeps

the door of his room open in order to talk with people who pass and tells
about his diarrhea and so on... Some days previously, he had told me
that he had gone to a barbecue house, had eaten a very good barbecue.
I began to think that he had intended to say that my mother was eatable,
was a kind of food, eatable, was eatable and that he, the guest, was the
owner of the barbecue house.

Bion: Why do you suppose he's telling you all this? What does he expect you to do about it?

A: To fill in the time. To fill in the session, the session time.

Bion: What for?

A: To flee from talking about his main difficulties or something.

Bion: Did you ask him why he was telling you?

A: No. Now, I remember that I more or less proposed him to go away and I could make him to accept the invitation of the cinematographer.

Bion: What do you feel the point is, that you want us to discuss with yourself?

A: My being afraid of having acted and being interested in the result, the result of my patient having some kind of work - not going on indefinitely treating with me.

Bion: So, your own impression is that you didn't do it right or catch it on the wrong length, or something.

A: I beg your pardon?

Bion: I was wondering why, or what, you expected us to say about this, or in what way can we help, do you think...?

A: I thought that, from this material, it could be possible for us to grasp some communication that remains meaningless to me, for me until now.

Bion: Yes, well now, can you focus down upon it a bit more... what is it that you feel is not clear to you, but which might be clear to us?

A: I think I could grasp the meaning of...
        [As the analyst hadn't understood what Dr. Bion was saying, a translator,
        at this point, explained in Portuguese what Dr. Bion was asking]
        I think that what is clear for me is that my material is producing sleep, sleep producing, because I saw you sleeping and nodding, this touched, this entered me, as an answer that my material is worthless.

Bion: Yes, but the point is: what is the point for you, as far as that's concerned? Why are you telling us this, about this. What do you think we can do about it?

A: If I start from the point, I just mentioned, I hope... or I am trying to understand what... disturbed my... work, my document, what is the result, of this? If, when I am talking, I can't receive any comments...

Bion: That concerns a supervision.

A: Yes.

Bion: It's of no interest whatever with regard to this patient. What is the point about the patient? What do you think we can say about this patient, which you yourself can't say?

A:	Ah, yes, yes! I think that with this session I intended to transmit the idea that this patient is with delusions...
Bion:	Yes. Now, what has made you think that this patient is deluded?
A:	The topics in which I could not link the words, or the phrases with the consequences, or with the conclusions.
Bion:	Can you give an example of that? What made you think that that was a sign that he was deluded?
A:	Once when he told me that, by hearing, by listening to the guest talk about the barbecue, the good barbecue, he immediately remembered or recalled, he was stricken by the idea that the guest was referring to his mother.
Bion:	Yes. Now, did you draw his attention to the fact that he seemed to think that that was the case and what did he expect you to do about it? Did you say: *"You are telling me this about the guest, but what am I to do? What am I, the analyst, to do about it?"*
A:	I did not.
Bion:	It is important to know what he thinks you can do about what he's telling you. Why is he? After all, I can understand that he thinks that you'll analyze him - if that's what he thinks. I can understand that he thinks you're set up to be a psychoanalyst, but what I'm not clear about is: what does he expect you as a psychoanalyst to do about it? Other than analyze you? Supposing he comes back now. What for? What are you supposed to do?
P1:	What is the importance – in every case is the same point of view – that we must know what the state of the patient was?
Bion:	Well, yes. But what has the patient said? What does the patient expect you to do?
P1:	We must know what is the theory of the patient, every moment?
Bion:	I would say: there I am, it's my working time and I'm setting up to be a psychoanalyst - that's fine! What's he come to see a psychoanalyst for? Why does he come to see me, during my working hours? I'd like to know.
P2:	I am thinking that, perhaps, he gets some problem of a counter-transference.
Bion:	Some?
A:	Some problem of counter-transference.
Bion:	That doesn't matter.
P2:	It doesn't matter.
Bion:	No, it doesn't matter! There is nothing that the analyst can do about counter-transference.
P2:	Yes, I understand that but... yes!...
	[Some words were lost in the change over]
A:	...he was analyzed in X, by one analyst name Dr. X...[10]
Bion:	Yes, that's all right!! But the question is: what does he expect you to do which his previous analyst hasn't already done?
A:	Yes. I think now that he expects from me, that I proceed with my relationship with him, in the same way we have...
Bion:	What makes you think that he expects that?

A: The good situation of receiving money from his relative.

Bion: That has nothing to do with you.

A: Yes.

Bion: I'm still giving it the point: what are you supposed to do?

A: I think that I am only supposed to analyze him, only this.

Bion: Yes, now how has he shown that?

A: He?

Bion: Um hum.

A: Remaining coming again and again.

Bion: But he might be coming again and again for analysis.

A: I think he is coming again for analysis.

Bion: Why do you think so?

A: Because...

Bion: That's what I'm getting at: what is the evidence to suggest he is coming again and again for analysis?

A: Because he thinks I'm an analyst! I think that I'm an analyst and, oh, he is suffering, he needs...

Bion: What's he suffering from?

A: He is suffering because he wishes to work and is not being able to work; because, of the complaint of not being accepted at the place where he...

Bion: Right! What does he expect you to do about that?

A: Yes, I think that he expects that I arrange some kind of work for him, though...

Bion: Did you tell him that he expected that? Did you point out to him that you are only a psychoanalyst; you're not an employment agency. If you were running an employment agency, you could say: *"Right, what can I do for you?"* Now, why hasn't he told you what he thinks you can do for him? Why has he come to you? Why is the analyst supposed to know what he wants?

A: Only by the patients...

Bion: Look: supposing I wanted a pair of shoes. I wouldn't go into a shoe shop and sit down and talk to him of my private life, I'd tell him: *"I want a pair of shoes"*. Now, why can't he tell you what he wants from you?

A: Because, I didn't ask him whether... I didn't tell him that he...

Bion: But, how can you? It's up to him to tell you what he wants. What are you to do for somebody who comes in and doesn't tell you what he wants?

A: Ask him what he wants, or tell the patient!

Bion: No, I'm sorry!! It seems to me that I can't be at all clear: what you think, that this patient thinks, you can do about it. All that I know is: you might try to analyze him, if he wanted analysis; but, if he doesn't tell you what he wants, then, I don't see what you can do about it.

A: He came because he was caught, by force, to a hospital at night and after...

P1:   A psychiatric hospital?

A: Yes!

Bion: He tells you this?

A: Yes.

Bion: Did you ask him, why he's coming to see you? Or what he thought you could do about the hospital?

A: About the hospital?

Bion: Did he tell you, what he thought you ought to do about the hospital?

A: I don't have anything to do with the hospital!

Bion: I don't mind about that! Does he go into a shoe shop and expect the shoe shop to do something about the going into a hospital?

  [Dr. Bion is now speaking very slowly and clearly in English, trying to make his point understood]

  Why then does he treat you differently?

A: I'm going...

Bion: Why does he pick on you and treat you differently from what he would treat a shoe shop?

A: Only if... I'm going beyond the shoes.

Bion: I don't really understand what you're doing. I don't understand why, if I say that I'm a psychoanalyst, somebody can't tell me what they want, or leave me to assume that what they want is for me to do analysis. Otherwise, why does he treat me in this special kind of way, which he doesn't treat shoe shops?

A: Yes! With these words, I clearly see that, because I didn't treat him as the patient.

Bion: That's alright, in a sense! I can see that you may have made this, or that, or the other mistake - we all do! What isn't so clear is: why he thinks that psychoanalysts should be treated differently from anybody else? It doesn't matter much as far as the patient is concerned; but you'll get other people and one would want to know: why such a person doesn't tell the analyst what he expects the analyst to do, or what he wants. Now, I know that we can make allowances for patients and we can think: *"Well, he is a very old man and he may not be able to do this"*; but, it doesn't alter the central point. I can say to him:

  Do you walk into such and such shop, or place, or person, or brother-in-law, or brother, or uncle and treat them in this particular way? Why do you treat me like this? I'm not your uncle, I'm not your brother or your sister or mother. I'm a mere psychoanalyst.

  Now, I could say to him:

  You have come here for some reason, what do you want? This is my consulting room, what do you expect me to do? Do you treat everybody like this? Or is this the special treatment that you reserve for me?

A: Now, the *"why"* is inside me, *why*? Why this patient, why is this person behaving so and so with me?

Bion: This idea of his being inside you and so on… is a psychoanalytic interpretation. This is a psychoanalytic theory. I don't object to that, what it doesn't answer is: what this patient wants and why he treats you, or me, or anybody else, in a special way? I don't know about how he treats the hotel manager, or anybody else, any more than you do; but, you do know something about how he treats you and you can ask him why he picks on you, to treat you in this particular way. Why does he expect you to make yourself available at, whatever the time is. Now, for example: is he expecting you to have an appointment which you're going to give him?

A: Only an appointment?

Bion: Well, I'm asking a question.

A: Yes, but, I think I couldn't grasp the meaning of your words.

Bion: Simply: is he expecting you to give him an appointment?

A: That way?

Bion: I don't know any other way… I don't know any other way of asking you the question, except: you know this patient and you know what arrangements you've made with him.

A: The arrangements I made with him, was to receive him to…

Bion: When?

A: Seven and a half years ago.

Bion: That doesn't matter! Don't mind what happened seven and a half years ago, I want to know what the arrangement is now.

A: Now?

Bion: Um hum.

A: Now, I advised him to go away, to work with that man.

Bion: Yes, that's alright! That is simply something which has been settled, but the point is: what do you expect to happen now, next? What's the next thing?

A: I think that I have the idea that he will go to work with the man and…

Bion: That's alright! But you don't know what he'll do and nor do I, nor does anybody else. You have told him something, you've given him advice. We don't know whether he'll pay the slightest attention to it, or what he'll do. But, what the question arises now is: what is the arrangement with him that you've made now?

A: To accept his attitude without analyzing it, or going more deeply into it.

Bion: But: why? Once you depart from your own particular job, we don't know what you've implied that you're prepared to do. In your own mind this is a good question for taking up with your analyst, or something of that sort. But, with regard to this particular man, the question is: what arrangement, what contract, so to speak, is there between you and him?

A: The temporary contract existing only to expect the letter contacting him to work, to be employed.

Bion: I don't see what that has to do with you. I can understand, that it is understood that he, if he wants an appointment with you, or wants an analysis, he'll write and ask you, or phone you, ask for an appointment. I can understand that. I can understand that you can profess to be an analyst, or a doctor, that you would actually treat him - if it was a physical illness or physical complaint - if he would tell you what he wants from you. I don't see what else you can do. You might say: *"No"*, that you are full up, or that you have other things to do, but what is the arrangement?

A: The arrangement, as you are saying, is up to me.

Bion: Right! Well, tell me then, what is the arrangement?

A: The arrangement is to propose a term and tell him that... or ask him first...
        [long silence]

P2:   I think that it is a false situation between him and his patient.

Bion: I think it is.

P2:   The first thing what that analyst must do, if he has the opportunity, is to...

P1:   Make clear!

P2:   ...make clear - clarify - what the patient wants from him, what is the expectative from the patient.

Bion: I think, otherwise, you seem to me to be letting yourself in for, like entering into an engagement in which one doesn't know what the terms of the contract are. But, if you are a psychoanalyst, if your working hours are - whatever they are - then you can say: *"Right, if you want an appointment from me, I can see you at such and such a time on"* - whatever the date is. But, it's up to him to tell you what he wants. You're not a blood relation of his, he's not your son, or wife or daughter...

A: Or father!

Bion: Yes, you're not a blood relation. As I understand it, all that you are doing is: you've made it known that if anybody wants an analysis, you are available between certain hours, but it's up to the patient to say what he wants.

A: May I ask you how should I ask the patient what he wants?

Bion: Just like that!

A: What?

Bion: What do you want? You could say: *"How did you come to come here?"* I wouldn't say but I could think and say: *"Well, I'm not a hotel treatment, I haven't got any rooms for rent. I'm not his uncle, I haven't got any money to pay for him to have an analysis or anything"*.

A: *"I am not a hospital!"*

Bion: No! Now, the question is, I could say to him: *"Do you ask anybody what you're asking me, or is this special?"*

A: This is a request?

Bion: Yes.

A: Yes, all this reminds me of my position, of my behavior.

Bion: I know, but your behavior and so on... are problems which you can take up with your analyst - whoever that might be - or you can leave alone. With this patient, the situation is different: all these matters of counter-transference and whatever your problems are... are nothing whatever to do with him.

A: You mean that I have not investigated, I had not asked directly to the patient what he wants?

Bion: It might have been no use if you had, I'm not saying that you should, but the point is this: it is important that the patient should explain why he thinks you should be treated differently from any other professional man, who has these professional hours. That you are prepared to put certain hours of the day aside for people who want analysis.

A: Yes.

Bion: When it comes to that you'll do your best. Now, supposing this patient wants - goodness knows what - you could simply say: *"I'm sorry, I am not a hotel keeper, I am not the director of the hospital. I'm only an analyst"*. Now, whether you say that or not is a matter of your own judgment. But it is as well to be quite clear in your own mind that that is all that you really proposed to do - there's nothing else that you can do!

A: I don't know what I said to him, to tell here. I frequently had ideas of telling him that the treatment is terminated, that I'm not the...

Bion: Yes. Well, you're raising quite a problem because one just has to face it: that this isn't the last time this will happen to you. If it was, one wouldn't bother about it. But, it's sure to happen again; so long as one is engaged in this kind of work, you're sure to meet this kind of person and it is well to be clear in your own mind where you draw the line. Now, I think all that the analyst can do is: to give such interpretation as he can do and all that one can expect from the patient is that the patient can say what he wants – what he's come for.

A: For me, this sounds so simple that it has been very, very difficult to see...

Bion: I know! It sounds terribly simple! I quite agree with you! And it is very surprising, in practice, if you try analysis, if you're set up as an analyst, to see what there is so difficult about them: what is so simple. In fact, there's a big difference here between: what appears to be a very simple thing and practicing this very simple thing.

A: From the very beginning?

Bion: Yes, always! One doesn't know when, any of us really, started being psychoanalysts: long before we ever heard of psychoanalysis, I'm sure.

A: Yes, from now.

Bion: You need to be quite clear whether you want to see this patient or not. Now, about that, you can say something: you can't say really anything much about the patient, but, you can say something about yourself and the sort of life you want to lead. So, it's important to get clear about this point of: what you are prepared to do and what you think you can do. There's very little that analysts can do. One can try to give interpretations, if anybody wants to listen to them and if anybody will tell you, or keep you properly informed. So, I think that however simple the base line must be, never mind about what other people can do and so on... You've got to say what you expect!

Notes

1 Editors' Note: From the tape, we gather that the analyst speaks in an at times almost incomprehensible English. Even though there was a translator present, he insisted in speaking directly to Dr. Bion and to the participants in English. This causes a confusion that is explicit throughout the session – a fact that added to the difficulty in transcribing the text from the tape. With apologies to our readers, we have tried to leave unaltered a sense of the 'roughness' of the discourse, assuming that this was part of the emotional turbulence brought into the supervision and that this may have been relevant to the *analytic* situation and certainly conveyed the experience of the supervisory encounter.

2 Editors' Note: Presumably, a student at the same school film that the patient had attended?

3 Editors' Note: Perhaps X refers to a specific role in film production: cinematographer, director, etc.

4 Editors' Note: Presumably, after discussing it with the analyst in session.

5 Editors' Note: is it an artifact of the translation and the wish to maintain anonymity for confidentiality purposes or is there some confusion as to who lives and goes where? Is this confusion a reflection of the analytic situation or the patient's mental state? Is the analyst's insistence on speaking a language that he can't communicate comprehensively in a reflection of something in the transference-countertransference of the treatment or the result of an unconscious projection communicated by the patient about his internal emotional state and therefore needing recognition and analytic clarification?

6 Editors' Note: The italics here and in the following pages indicates that it is the patient who is talking.

7 Editors' Note: There is a confusion that seems to enter the supervisory discussion at this point. The 'he' Bion seems to be asking about – "When he complained of the other guest?" – would seem to refer to the patient. But the analyst seems to misunderstand this and responds as if the 'he' refers to the owner of the hotel. Again, to what extent is this an artifact of translation and transcription or is it a turbulence and confusion being projected into the supervision, because it represents something that needs to be unconsciously expressed, recognized and addressed?

8 Editors' Note: Even though the next line is in italics, it is unclear if it was the analyst's intervention, or the patient's. Could this 'editorial error' be still another signal of self/object confusion? And then could Bion's wish to 'close the window' and 'turn off the noise', in addition to being a true architectural issue of literal fact, reflect a wish to shut down the chaos that is building and being conveyed? Later it will turn out that the patient had some idea that the 'disturbing guest' thought that the patient's mother was 'eatable', so perhaps it is the patient talking here.

9 Editors' Note: Although in italics, this last statement is not in quotes and so leaves open the question of whether it was the patient's association or the analyst's intuition. The italics resume in the next sentence: "This guest is really unbearable to me …" and from the context it is the patient speaking.

10 Editors' Note: There is a problem in transcription of the tape, but it may be that they are talking about a previous attempt at analysis in the patient's home state.

Supervision D10 commentary

Evelise de Souza Marra

In clinical practice as described by Freud, Klein and Bion, whom I see as a continuous series of authors, a process of gradual but substantial change took place as we passed from one set of functions for the analyst, into another. That is, we almost inadvertently ceased to interpret the unconscious, identify anxieties and their corresponding defenses, separate the external and internal worlds and separate reality from fantasy. Gradually the role of analysts evolved into participation in the emotional experiences that occur in the analytic sessions. In this situation, analysts, in contact with their transformations, are subject to the emotional turbulence inherent to this experience. Under these conditions, one hopes that formulations in knowledge (transformations in K) appropriated to the analyst can evolve, in the analysand, from knowing to being (transformations in O).

As a result, descriptions became operational, although Bion himself continued to use the term 'interpretation' to refer to interventions by analysts in their clinical work. He recommended that analysts should center their work on the emotional experience taking place, which has an origin (O) that is common to both participants, albeit unknowable. Clinical work is guided by the assurance that, despite the turbulence, there can be mental growth (development of the alpha function). Bion's emphasis is on the evolution from Knowing to Being and on the evolution of the unknown of mental reality. He also held that both analyst and analysand are affected. In Bion, the notion of faith in the encounter as the possibility for advances into the unknown and into the truth about one's self is a central part of the psychoanalytic preconception.

It should also be stressed that, for Bion, 'thinking' occupied the center of analytic work to the point that some of his readers have raised the question as to the place of sexuality in his work. Our understanding is that sexuality and thought are fused together in his theory of thinking, centralized in the development of the alpha function and in the ideographic expression ($♀♂$) relative to projective identification, reverie and the relationship between container and contained. But it is the genesis and use of thinking that gradually occupied analysts, together with the proposition of examining the myth of Oedipus with its central element being the crime of his arrogance in seeking the truth at any cost.

DOI: 10.4324/9781003439233-9

These expansions had far-reaching repercussions in clinical practice and extend as well to the activity traditionally known as 'supervision'. I see supervision as an experience where an analyst presents herself or himself to another analyst through memories (and new associations) of an episode experienced with a 'patient' at some earlier time in some other place. The analyst who takes on the function of supervisor only has direct access to the analyst who is presenting the case, while the 'patient' being focused on becomes present solely through the experience of this analyst being supervised.

It seems to me that without our having developed a theory of technique for this type of encounter – and we have not even done so for clinical work itself – analysts being supervised gradually kept the focus on their patients while the supervising analyst concentrated on the analyst with whom he was going through the experience. We saw changes in practice before a theory of technique was developed that could support the incredible passage implied in Bion's suggestion to replace the dyad of *conscious and unconscious* with *finite and infinite*, and to place the theory of the alpha function as the center of thinking and emotion. It seems to me that this Supervision (D10), conducted by Bion, clearly illustrates this and it is here that I would like to concentrate my arguments. I am interested in what we do as analysts, supervisors or persons being supervised, using these terms (*supervision, supervisor, analyst being supervised*) only because we have not yet created any others that can take into account the expansions we are discussing.

At the beginning of Supervision D10 Bion asks: "What does the patient want and what does the analyst think he, the analyst, can do?" Bion says that the analyst should pay attention to how the patient treats him or her, and farther ahead he specifies the question and asks: "**What do you think** this patient wants of you?" "Why do you think he is telling you all these things?" "What does he expect you to do about this?"

I also call attention to the following aspects:

1   Bion asked the analyst being supervised: "What do you want from me?" "Do you think you did something wrong and that we know what would be right?" "Do you think that what is unclear for you is clear for us?"
2   What 'evidence' do you have that the analysand is repeatedly coming to analysis?
3   What agreement is there between you? Not that of the beginning, but that right now?
4   What can you do as a 'psychoanalyst'?
5   He also calls attention to interest in the unknown (he said, "The important thing is what is ahead"); he says that it is all very simple, or seems simple, but in fact is very difficult.
6   There is also his reference to counter-transference as that with which there is nothing to do, because it deals with the analysis of the analyst.
7   Finally, we have emphasis on "what is of interest in relation to this patient"; that is, what is important in analysis is the question "what is of interest in this patient"?

It seems to me that Bion invites the analyst to 'think'. The analyst should think about how he sees and relates with this patient, about what the function of each member of the dyad is, what the expectations are and what agreement has been made between them. At the same time that he does this with the analyst under supervision, Bion tries to identify what the analyst wants from him and from the group, and he does this through direct questions. He indicates a method at the same time that he carries it out. It seems to me that the climate of emotional turbulence and the difficulties with language are 'evident'.

Therefore I call special attention to the focus on thinking, rather than on seeking out or interpreting unconscious contents. To Bion's first question the analyst answers with the theory of the unconscious, and the theory of anxiety and defenses, when he interprets that "the patient fills in the time in order to escape from his difficulties". But Bion insisted on the theory of thinking when he asked the analyst, "Did you ask why [the patient] was saying this to you?" "And what do you want us to discuss with you?"

For my purposes here I might mention the reference to 'evidence' in psychoanalysis and the reference as to what analysis and psychoanalytic inference are ("What would you as an analyst say to this patient?"). In regard to this point I remember Bion's article entitled *Evidence* (1976), published two years after this supervision; it could serve as a reference for some of the theoretical questions of the technique in construction.

In the article, we have the example, which was never clear to me, of the reference by the patient to the "memory of the parents at the upper part of Y-shaped stairs". Bion associates to 'Why-shaped stare' and he dreams, or imagines, starting with the visual image of the letter Y, of a cone spatially projected toward the outside and a breast (a point) projected toward the inside. In other words, he makes a connection with the primal scene and the Oedipal situation. In the following session he 'gives an interpretation', which he does not specify in the article, suggesting that the patient had made some visual slip, or exchange. The analysand agrees with Bion's comment that, "It took a few seconds, didn't it?" And they share the evidence of the double meaning or a single meaning. Despite the agreement, Bion stresses that it was impossible to know what the evidence was for the patient and what it was for the analyst. Although I did not easily catch the play on words, I noted the recommendation and the difficulties concerning the evidence of our psychoanalytic conjectures, observations, feelings, perceptions and interpretations. This holds true both in analysis and in what we call supervision.

To pinpoint the nature of the problem, Bion talks about the need to observe in a state of emptiness until something makes sense (a recommendation that Charcot passed on to Freud many years before). Bion brings up the apparent caesura between prenatal and natal, and between primitive and organized in terms of the mental world. He reminds us that, in psychoanalysis, we allow ourselves to use feelings like facts and we should develop our own language and master it. He also considers that what goes on in the analyst's mind has to do with the patient's mind (an act of faith).

Evidence brings up essential questions related to technique, as well as "How to make the best of a bad deal", "Emotional turbulence", "Catastrophic change" and "Caesura". But a "theory of technique" is still an open question, a development that would coherently bring together theory and practice with the developments of the theory of thinking in Bion. His contributions and way of communicating, more than ever, brought psychoanalysis closer to theories of complexity, that is, closer to the principles of the uncertainty, incompleteness, and undecipherability of one's origin, namely, infinity, singularity and negativity, in the words of Arnaldo Chuster in *A Psicanálise: Dos princípios ético-estéticos à clínica* [*Psychoanalysis: From ethical and aesthetic principles to the clinic*].

In supervision D10 we again come across the question of 'psychoanalytic' formulation or action. For Bion our focus is on the personality or character of the analysand and, therefore, things are not taking place in the aseptic atmosphere of a laboratory but in live contact with us. What, then, engages our personality (conscious and unconscious, primitive and thinking, known and unknown) in the emotional turbulence inherent in the encounter between two minds. In this context, what do we do or what can we do as analysts? The answer is surely to analyze, which may sound easy, but in practice it is quite difficult.

What does the analyst of the 'emotional experience' analyze? What is this experience that brings about slow and fleeting transformations in K that will be useful if transformed into O, but that fail to attain what the analyst values, that is, the unknown, the coming-to-be? What does he analyze in the conception of a discipline where the ineffable, the unspeakable and the impossibility of indicating origins escape at every moment? What does he analyze, being aware that his thinking is organized in the possible dream-imagination of his observations?

I believe that analysts can only analyze according to their own references, namely, the theories about mental functioning that have made some sense to them and their so-called 'weak theories' without scientific status but from which they derive their values in life, their personal myths, their family ties, their personality and their potential. But analysts should essentially remain in a state of questioning, or a state devoid of certainties, 'without memory and without desire', with faith that 'something speaks' or 'feels' or 'thinks'. Then, perhaps, analysts will move closer to finding a successful language (a language of achievement) in which to address the evolving O of the moment.

For Bion, in accordance with his method, I see that the sessions both with patients and with supervisees are opportunities to focus on the nature of this problem in order to continue dealing with it.

Chapter 5

Supervision D4

Bion: To go on where we left off.[1] Well, I was suggesting it's a problem giving an interpretation to the patient, to the analysand, which was really addressed to a particular aspect of his statement, because one listens to the statement that the patients makes, but one is also observing what we consider to be the personality. I don't know what one is to call that, or in what way one would satisfy the scientist if you said: what is a personality? I don't think it is very satisfactory to look the verb up in a dictionary and this is one of the difficulties about this whole matter that we are talking about. For example, a patient talks quite freely and quite easily, he says he doesn't have dreams and he has no imagination. But, for month after month, while he comes to every session, never fails, never has an illness. doesn't catch colds, when he gets on to the couch at first, he seems to have got difficulty, about which, I didn't bother very much, because it appeared to be simply a question of adjusting his clothes and a discomfort on the couch. But, after about three months I thought this was very peculiar. He always lay in a slightly awkward position on the couch, and when he lays down, he'd lie like that and then he'd raise his head like that,

[at this point Dr. Bion was, obviously, making signs with his hands]

as if he were struggling against some sort of opposition and trying to see his feet. He did that three or four times and I hadn't the faintest idea what he was doing, or even how to tell myself what that peculiar movement was. He was so co-operative, so rational and I was kept very well informed.

He said that he only slept an hour or two each night, and he used to work for about sixteen hours a day, for seven days a week. The only holidays he took were when I had a break. There was no complaint about it, no disturbance, no depression. When other patients are used to having some kind of reaction to the fact that I was stopping, we could break all the same! Now, all right! I thought that I would change my vertex, because I thought that I obviously couldn't see anything very much from where I was looking or observing this patient. But, when I did that it occurred to me that his precise and exact position on the couch could be comprehensible if he were lying of the edge of a precipice and then, his position, his

DOI: 10.4324/9781003439233-10

posture, began to look very much like a cataleptic attitude and the whole analysis began to look like a sort of compulsive ritual. The same hour, the same behaviour, no diversion from that position at all and the more I saw of him, the more I felt that these were not ordinary communications and then my interpretations themselves fitted into the pattern – I wondered what kind of psychiatric diagnosis one would make. I thought that the nearest I could get to it would be that the total situation in the consulting room could be a *"follies a deux"*. So that one could certainly claim a part in this relationship.

Then, I began to look at and listen to the behaviour of *both* these people, one of whom was myself! I continued giving what I considered to be psychoanalytic interpretations, continued to observe, listen in to that peculiar conversation; it fitted very well what I've been used to calling the free association and the interpretations they fitted in beautifully. You can call it the marriage of two minds, but there was something wrong with it. It wasn't exactly *homosexual*, you couldn't call it heterosexual. In fact, you couldn't call it sexual at all, not if the word sex means the kind of thing that it means in botany or physiology, or what I would call psychoanalysis. But, I imagine to effect some change in this, because as that pattern became clear to me, I felt I could make it clear to the patient and I found a formulation or at least a number of formulations, which seemed to make it comprehensible to the patient, that I had departed from him.

Then, it appeared that this same relationship existed between him and somebody else. that I also interpreted, when it got clear to me that the deficiency had been made good by his being able to enlist the co-operation of some other member of the public, with which he had a social relationship. So that, I also interpreted. Again a change occurred, after some time, I may say, and now, he fell back onto having the same sort of relationship with himself. So, I interpreted that, but after a time I wondered what this self was. What does it mean himself? Herself? Myself? What is this self?

I find it most unsatisfactory the thought about his body and his mind, because both those words have quite a large order of meaning. The body is a thing that you take to your physician. The mind, you didn't bother with; and indeed, if one talked about his mind, if I was talking about some quite insupportable conviction like: talking about God to an atheist and the same thing would apply to any of the various gods which have existed. The kind of gods that are mentioned in classical literature or in Homer. I was not sure of this bit, because it was devoid of live-looking, devoid of content. Well, I tried getting it in location, I talked about his feelings and the sort of thing that he did up here.

[Dr. Bion made a gesture here no doubt pointing to his head]

It was clear that he didn't understand what I meant, or thought it was just nonsense, anyway. But he was quite polite, he didn't say that. He certainly ignored any reference to up here or down there

[again Dr. Bion made a gesture at this point]

or anything of that sort, so I'm thrown back on still talking about himself and sometimes I said: *"Now you're talking as if yourself was located in your spleen."*

I really didn't know quite what to say to him, sometimes I would have said that it was located in his kidneys.[2] I didn't have to, because, after a time he talked about people who ran away or people who were very aggressive and what I would say? *"This person that you say runs away and this person that you say is very impressive, they're the same person. I think that they're yourself".* Now, the same peculiar mobility became more and more pronounced. I had to go on chasing this self around what seems to be various areas, of what I had been taught was anatomy. Well, I won't continue the story because, it extended from there

[another gesture must have been made]

and it became evident that the self was not within the limits of what I called his body. So, I had to extend my interpretations over an area that had different boundaries and indeed, it became clearer that it hadn't got any boundaries. In order to express it at all, I'd have to borrow a term like *infinity*.

It reminded me very much of the words of Milton,[3] which might express it very well when he talks about: *"Won from the void and formless infinite"*. In the Introduction to the Third Book, there are a number of very expressive formulations. He talks about being *"long detained in that obscure [sojourn]"*. And he speaks about outer and inner darkness and the middle darkness: *"And up to reascend though hard and rare"*.[4] That would seem to me to be a very good description of this patient if he had descended into what psychoanalysts call the unconscious and remained there a very long time: *"Though long detained in that obscure sojourn and up to reascend"*, as if that was something very unusual. But when he does reascend instead of emerging in the world of light, he finds himself blinded. Now Melanie Klein gave me an interpretation which puzzled me for a long time she said: *"You feel mutilated castrated, as you emerge from the womb"*.[5]

[....] That called REM (Rapid Eye Movement). Before that, I think that when he says he had a dream, met so and so and was very annoyed with him and so on... I think in fact he did and I think he'd be extremely rude. I happen to know that, because that same person, of whom he'd dreamt, came to me for analysis

[a burst of laughter from the audience]

So, I heard that story.

[Someone in the background makes a comment]

to which Dr. Bion says: *"Yes"*

[then he goes on]

from the person, that the patient that I'm talking about, dreamt. Well, I shall be very glad to hear what language you think I ought to talk to this patient and what I should say to him if I know that language. It's clear that the language he was talking was extremely accurate. His statements were really reliable.[6] I could rely on his statements as easily as I could rely on his coming to the consulting room with such accuracy that I could put my watch right by him. There's no question about his being late; my watch might be fast or slow, but not him! I don't know what clock he was going by, but it was right! So, in fact, I can't tell you anything about how to analyse that patient. So, I hope you'll be able to tell me something.

[At this point the tape recorded was switched off for a second; then we hear a woman's voice saying]

P1:   ... memory and ... memory and ...

P2:   Intuition!

P1:   Intuition, and what do you think about the thought without the thinker?

Bion: To take the last point first, I would suggest that we imagine that when a number of people collect together, like this, there are stray thoughts floating around, trying to find a mind to settle in. So, the problem from the point of each individual – each one of us – is: can we catch one of these wild thoughts without being too particular about what race they are or what category they are? Whether they are memories or intuitions! But, just get hold of any one of these wild thoughts however strange or however savage or friendly they might be. Give it a home and then allow it to escape from your lungs; in other words, give it birth, no matter how wild the idea may be.

Notes

1 Editor's Note: The nature of the previous discussion referred to here is unclear from the transcript and recording. However, Bion here is, and perhaps had been before, talking of a patient of his own.

2 Transcriber's Footnote: See paragraph above where he speaks of Homer's location of the mind. On the other hand, Dr. Bion repeats ad nauseum this story of where the mind is located: in the spleen, in the diaphragm, in the kidneys, etc.

3 Editor's Note: Bion is referring to Milton's *Paradise Lost.*

4 Editor's Note: Bion is quoting from the following passage:
"Before the Heavens thou wert, and at the voice
Of God, as with a Mantle didst invest
The rising world of waters dark and deep,
Won from the void and formless infinite".
Thee I re-visit now with bolder wing,
Escap't the *Stygian* Pool, though long detain'd
In that obscure sojourn, while in my flight
Through utter and through middle darkness borne
With other notes then to th' *Orphean* Lyre
Isung of *Chaos* and *Eternal Night*,
Taught by the heav'nly Muse to venture down
The dark descent, and up to reascend,
Though hard and rare:"

5 Editor's Note: Unfortunately, there is a break here and the rest of Bion's commentary about this patient is lost.

6 Transcriber's Footnote: In another supervision in a different context, Bion says exactly the opposite.

Supervision D4 commentary
Entering and leaving the mine

Ruggero Levy

As always, Bion makes us think. The text in this supervision is like a mine of precious stones. At first, all is dark. You can't see much. Gradually, however, it lights up, and then there are treasures to explore. I will begin this text by giving an overview of Bion's supervision, which has undergone a number of transformations until arriving at its current form in Portuguese, so that afterwards we can extract some of its riches. Certainly, much will remain hidden in the text/mine, waiting for another miner to come along.

Initially, Bion introduces the problem of interpretation: on the one hand, it is directed to what the patient says, his statements; on the other, however, we are simultaneously with the patient in the analysis room, observing what he does, receiving other forms of communication, being affected by his postures, gestures, tone of voice, etc. Which of these is to be addressed?

Thus speech, or discourse, is a part of the patient's personality, but everything else, *the "void, formless and infinite"* is also there.

But, then again, what is the personality?

Bion discusses the case of a patient who speaks freely, but does not dream, and has no imagination. He remarks that some of the patient's bodily attitudes on the couch initially seemed meaningless, but then he realizes there is something peculiar about them. However, in parallel, he felt well informed by the patient's discourse; the patient was quite 'cooperative'. But – the patient could not sleep. He never slept more than an hour or two each night!

Bion then thought he should observe his patient from another vertex. And from this other vertex, what seemed to be an innocent movement of the head to peer at the feet was imagined by Bion as the posture of someone standing on the edge of a precipice. And in this light, the patient's sessions began to seem like a compulsive ritual. Bion thought these were not ordinary communications, and so he adjusted his interpretations to them. He does not tell us exactly what his interpretations were but implies that if someone had entered the room, they would have certainly thought it was a *folie à deux*.

He went on to yet another vertex and began to observe the pair as if he were not a member of it. He had the impression that some of the patient's free associations and

DOI: 10.4324/9781003439233-11

his own interpretations fit together. Bion said that when he realized what was going on, he made some formulations that must have enabled the patient to understand that the analyst had, at that point, diverged from him. It also occurred to Bion that the patient had previously had a similar relationship with someone else outside the analytic setting, and this was also interpreted. That is, Bion seemed to understand and tell the patient that something good had happened there, while reproducing this relationship in the analysis.

But from that point, I understand that there was yet another change, with the patient resuming a relationship with himself. This is also interpreted. Then Bion starts asking: Which self is this? What is the self? And he imagines that asking the patient such questions would be like talking with an atheist about God, for the self was something that in the patient seemed to have no apparent life, no content. Bion tried, nonetheless, to determine its location: Where was the self? The patient either did not understand the question or thought it was ridiculous; however, being polite, he said nothing.

Bion then made conjectures – which he shared with the patient – regarding the location of the patient's mind. Where could it be? In the spleen, in the kidneys? The patient mentions people who flee and who are aggressive. Bion directly interprets that he, the patient, is, at the same time, all of these people. But the patient returns to his bodily movements and Bion understands that he would have to continue pursuing this elusive self. He then realizes that the self was not within the limits of the body and that his interpretations would have to be extended to an area that had different limits, or no limits, perhaps an infinite area. He mentions Milton – although it is not explicit in the text. I believe he meant the following passage from Book III of *Paradise Lost*: "The rising world of waters dark and deep, Won from the void and formless infinite" (Quoted in *Transformations*, p. 162).[1] He conjectures that it would be as if his patient had plunged into the infinite and formless darkness of his unconscious and emerged, not in a halo of light, but in blindness.

The text then follows with what would appear to be a sequence of questions and answers. In one of them, Bion refers to the wild thoughts that leap out of the mind and that, if sheltered without prejudice or restrictions, can be born and develop. And I think that, throughout the text, that is exactly what Bion does. He has an absurd ability to 'give a home' to wild thoughts, thoughts without a thinker. Although this seemed at times almost psychotic, it was actually courageous: he was unafraid to go crazy and think what was unthinkable to the patient – and perhaps to many of us. In a peculiar way, this supervision shows us how these thoughts, by not having a thinker, can still inhabit the lung or the spleen. However, the courage to give them 'a home', a container, can give them life and finally make them thinkable.

While reading and writing my own text I have made several associations. First, I was strongly reminded of Bion's book *Transformations*, because it also addresses the finality of interpretation. Bion says that the function of interpretation is to help the patient become himself, become 'O' But the patient resists by producing column 2 elements[2] due to the difficulty or impossibility of encountering his own emotions. This poses a dilemma for the analysis, since the patient resists becoming himself and can lead the analyst to also produce false statements. At the most, the patient *learns about* himself without *becoming* himself.

It seems to me that this is what Bion is talking about at the beginning of this supervision: that the punctual, cooperative, and polite patient could not become himself and these wild thoughts, located who knows where in the dark and formless infinity of his unconscious, prevented him from sleeping. The patient did not sleep. He could not dream his thoughts, his emotional life was impoverished, apparently plagued by many undigested facts. Bion, then, with the courage of a tank commander, realizes that he should be able to look at his patient from another vertex; Bion becomes the patient and seems to enter a world that an observer would say is a *folie à deux*. He imagines the patient standing at the edge of a precipice and understands his anguish at the possibility of falling into the void without form. But from then on, Bion felt in touch with and extremely close to his patient. I have the impression that perhaps at this point in the session Bion is capable of being *at one* with his patient and make transformations in K. He understands that the patient was fleeing from himself, perhaps because he could not bear to draw nigh to the infinite darkness of his mind. That is, he fled from himself and interpretations that could promote transformations in O, which he highly feared.

However, this discourse also brought to my mind Bion's 1976 paper "Evidence", in which he addresses the question of the depth and primitivism of the unconscious and the great dilemma in psychoanalysis of how to communicate with someone that is 'not I'. He discussed the lack of evidence that we are actually communicating with our patients, and reports a dramatic experience in which he believed he had been succeeding with a patient, but after the session the patient went home and committed suicide. He emphasized the difficulty of producing utterances, forging words that remain in good working order and do not grow smooth and worn like old coins. He alerts us to our tendency of filling in *the void of our terrifying ignorance* with proximate, portable paramnesias, which are the most familiar theories we carry. He then formulates one of his brilliant dictums: *there is an inexhaustible fund of ignorance to draw upon – it is about all we do have to draw upon.*[3] It is brilliant because if we want to come into contact with the dark and formless infinity of the unconscious, we must be able to immerse ourselves in it, to seek *to become it*, and then, only then, to know it. Finally, in Evidence, Bion warns us that we may be dealing with phenomena so subtle that they are almost imperceptible, but that are so real that they can destroy both us and our patients.

To conclude, being with Bion, thinking with him, thinking about him, always helps us become a little better as analysts, and we emerge from the mine with a few more precious nuggets. For all that, I am grateful for being here.

Notes

1 Bion, WR. *Transformations: Change from learning to growth.* London: Heinemann Medical Books, Ltd. 1965.
2 Column 2 of Bion's Grid is often associated with defensive operations and the negation of truth.
3 Bion, *Clinical seminars and other works*, p. 317.

Chapter 6

Supervision D6

T: The patient is forty-eight years old, and has been two times in analysis before. He's had ten years of experience of analysis before he came to Dr. X. He's been in analysis with him two and a half years. He's a descendent from the Brazilian, how do you say, noble family.

P1:   Ancestors.

T: Ancestors.

Bion: Yes, yes!

T: He was apparently rich, now he's very poor.

Bion: Did he tell you that he had had analysis before?

A: Yes. He did.

Bion: Yes! Did you say anything about that? Did you reply, interpret it to him?

A: I don't remember.

Bion: No! It's liable to happen quite a lot either you are dealing with people who have so little contact with analysis that they haven't been before, or they have been before and you get that kind of problem. Now, did he tell you that he had had analysis before?

A: Yes he did.

Bion: Yes! Did you say anything about that? Did you try to interpret it again?

A: I don't remember!

Bion: Now, suppose it's the first interview that you have with the patient and the patient tells you this. You could point out that from what they know about psychoanalysis, they would seem to have no particular reason for coming for some more psychoanalysis, knowing what they know about themselves and knowing what they know about psychoanalysis. So, one of the questions would be: what are they expecting you, the analyst, to say which they don't already know?

A: Yes, I understand.

Bion: Not to put them off, but to point out that there is a question here, which we don't know, but can guess. One could say: *"You've told me your feelings that you want to be somebody else. You want me to help you to be somebody else"*. Now, the same thing could apply even if he had been to you. You could say:

DOI: 10.4324/9781003439233-12

Although you've been to me for analysis before, you are still feeling that I could say something that I haven't said and you could get something from me that you haven't got, we don't know why you think that I could tell you something that I haven't already told you.

A: He wants a miracle…

Bion: After all, what made you think he wanted a miracle? Be inclined to say: *"Well, somebody was expecting a miracle. So, if it's clear that either you or I, or both, expect a miracle and neither you or I, or both of us, expect to reach a mere human being here".*

P1:   Pardon? Expect to?

Bion: Meet a mere human being.

So, in that case it doesn't sound that you thought you are likely to be expecting to meet just another person like you, or another person just like me. It sounds as if one of us, or both, expected to meet a kind of God, but even God can't be expected to obey the laws of nature.

For some reason, there is a belief, or an expectation, that God wouldn't obey the rules or the laws of the universe, or the world, as we know it. The laws of origin perhaps, but one doesn't know what this expectation is, or what kind of universe or world we live in. It does not obey the laws of nature, or, say, what one might call the laws of science; this is one of the reasons why, I think, psychoanalysts, all of us, are leaving out a very great deal of matters that we ought to consider.

We ought to know something about Religion. We ought to know something about Science. We ought to know something about Art. If that, pretty well, covers the ground, which in primitive terms, that more or less means the whole of the way human beings think, but it would also explain something else. I could say to a patient:

You, the analysand, must be coming here because you like being analyzed and want more analysis, or that, you like science and want more scientific explanations, or like art and want me or you to be more artistic. However, it is difficult to see why you saw who – it was – or you saw me before and why you've come back again to day.

Say:

When you tell me that you haven't got enough money, I think that this is something of a rationalization. Now, when I say rationalization, I don't mean that what you are saying isn't reasonable. On the contrary, I mean that it is reasonable, or it wouldn't be a rationalization; indeed, the reason, so to speak, for having a reason is to make things seem reasonable. So, if you are wanting miracles, you are also wanting me, or you, or both, to make a miracle reasonable. Now, I think that you must be afraid that you have not got – whatever you need – and that I haven't got whatever I need to make a miracle reasonable, or to make an ordinary, real thing, miraculous. In other words, you must be feeling that you and probably I are incapable of admiring being miraculous. So, there is a fear that neither you nor I are capable of admiring miracles; but, neither you nor I are capable of admiring facts; that neither you nor I are capable of admiring art. In short, it's not only money that you feel that you haven't got, that I haven't got, that nobody has got, whatever it needs to pay for analysis, whether it's money or knowledge, or artistic capacity or religious capacity, to be able to do what we want. There must be something that makes it possible for you to be here and for me to be here – two people in this same room.

A: And when I make …

Bion: *"In addition to what I've already said, you hope that what we can now call sex, would make the miracle possible. You hope that what we can now call religion could make sex religiously respectable; but the point is: there's a feeling that if you are being scientific, then it is not being in accordance with the rules of religion; if you're being religious, it is not in accordance with the rules of science. In short, whatever you are being, or I am being, it will be wrong".*

       There's always the other, what I call, the vertex. The advantage of using a term like vertex is it doesn't say… it doesn't mean anything. It's a variable, you can put in what you like. You can say: "If you've come here for a religious experience, then you'll only get a scientific or artistic one; if you've come here for the aesthetic experience or the scientific experience, you'll only get a religious one". In other words, whatever one does here will be wrong, whatever you expect here, will be, also, what you don't want.

A: May I ask you a question?

Bion: Can't be God, but if you are God, then there's a feeling God will be opposed to science, or the laws of nature and must object to the laws – whatever they are – which is obeyed by the world, or reality. He would have to know what the laws are which are obeyed by God. In short, who is God's God?

P: He would like to …

Bion: Remind him of what he has said and what he is doing now, as it were, in the actual session. Suppose this was the session, we're heading somewhere here, what is he doing, or expecting now, which he wouldn't get? Today is Sunday, what does he expect, today, which is different from what he expected yesterday? Or tomorrow? What is he wanting? Now, the further question is: we can say that here, we can do that here, but what are we to say supposing the patient is here, can we say, what should be said to this patient? And in what language? You can say: *"What you are telling me now reminds me of things that you've said before, such as"* – then, you might mention one or two.

*See, in this way, you are still today expecting to get from me something like what you have expected before. In other words, your expectation is still in the distance and it has still got a long history. It's a **preconception** and if*

*you think it's correct, I think you feel that you've seen me before and you
expect me to be rather like what I was last time.*

A: Always the same?

Bion: It's enough to think that this is the same person, there's something about
him and something about me, which one feels means that the person –
although they've changed – they've also like what they were before, that is
the constant [i.e., invariant].

It might be important to mention, or it might not. You might need to remind the patient that he thinks, or he feels, or he is the same and he thinks
that the analyst is the same or very similar. I think that I would say about this:

*Although in some ways you are not who you used to be and I am a differ-
ent person, even your own home is not your father's and mother's home,
you are feeling as if coming to analysis is going back to being a child and
being under the rule of a parent, although I'm not your father or mother
and you are not a child. The same thing, I think, applies probably to your
home, which reminds you of your first home. It wasn't your home but really
was your father and mother's home, but even then, I think that you thought
it was your home. What makes you think that? What is the evidence which
suggests to you that that is the case? Talking as if?*

A: And talking as if, yes, but that makes me [....]

Bion: You would need to know what your evidence was for saying that. I'm not
disagreeing with you, no! But I'm pointing out that it would be useful to
know what the evidence is, if you knew what the evidence was, then it
would be useful if you thought he could understand your obstinance. In
other words, it's necessary that you should know what the evidence is –
that's why he's got to come to you. The time to give that interpretation
hasn't arrived, because you know the interpretation.

P1:   Because she knows the interpretation?

Bion: Yes.

P1:   But she hasn't the evidence [....]

Bion: She's got to have the evidence – even if, she has.

P1:   Yes.

Bion: She ought really, I think, to wait; so that the analysand could understand
what she's talking about.

A: Can get [....]

Bion: *"I have the evidence of this and I think I can point this out to you, that you,
if you pay attention to what I'm saying, could also see this evidence".*

A: Which means that I can [....]

Bion: Really, it's no good telling children, say, about sex, without knowing what
is known to you, as a father or a mother, unless they can understand what
you are talking about. Now, the question is: when and what are you to tell
children? Even if you know about sex, when are you to tell them? If you

tell them anything about it, suppose you say: *"I won't tell them"*, then, somebody else will. Other children will and other children may not know enough about sex to tell your boy or girl about sex. On the other hand, you, as the father or mother, know more than the child could understand. So, one doesn't withhold information, but one doesn't give information which is incomprehensible. In fact, it is very difficult to know when to tell, say to children, anything about sex; because, if you don't, then it is to dictate. If you say: *"Don't do that"*, that's a dictate, but it's also a dictate if you give them an explanation, which they can't understand. Since they can't understand the explanation, it's a dictate. Now, it's not the same in analysis, but it is not dissimilar. None of us, if we're honest, really know much about psychoanalysis.

P: Now I understand why this patient sometimes accuses me [....]

Bion: Well, the advantage of analysis is that you can feel things; here whatever the advantages are of supervision, you haven't got that advantage of the analysis, practical analysis, but practical analysis you can feel, so can the patient.

P: [The participant asks a question about the patient and evidence].

Bion: But you must point out the evidence. You must point out:

If you were a small boy or a small girl and you were living in my house, in my consulting room, or if I were living in yours, it would be much easier to understand how you feel that there would be the feeling that somebody was father or mother, or even in the world in which you and I live, there is a father and mother. But, this father and mother appears to be one which doesn't obey the laws of science, doesn't obey the laws of the physical world. Who, or what, then, has invented, or created, or said what are the laws of science? Who, or what, has said are the laws of painting? Who said you've got to paint a picture of a house like this and who has told God what he's got to do?

P: [the intervention here was not clear on the tape but involved the word, 'precipitate'. Perhaps precipitate an argument or struggle?]

Bion: Can you give me an example? The point is this that precipitate is just one word, it's like 'omnipotent' or 'sex'. Freud increasingly and indeed, in his paper in 1937 I think, talked... but, he didn't think it was a question of using interpretations, in the sense of some words, but constructions, or as I would put it, it's no good saying precipitate to me, can you tell me a story? If I tell you a story, then you will understand what I mean when I say precipitate. But, let's imagine that the child or the patient wants to be told something like: how do you make babies? Now then, how do you say: you will have to wait until you are older, before I tell you how to do that, because...

        [end of side one of tape; some words were lost]

        ... I myself wouldn't bother about that very much. It may be wrong, but I feel that, to say quite rightly, that the patient is precipitating and so on...

it sounds like getting into an argument. *"You are precipitating". "No, I am right, you are wrong!" "No, you are wrong, I am right"*, it's endless.

P: No, it's not…

Bion: It shouldn't be! That's why it's no good giving that kind of interpretation. [….] the analyst is wrong.

A: The analyst is wrong?

Bion: No, I'm asking the question.

P1:   Do you say [….]

Bion: The question isn't whether this is correct or not, but what has the patient been told? The trouble with that is that…

[someone talking in Portuguese blocks out Dr. Bion's voice]

…in thinking that he could understand. Now, if he did understand, then it would be alright to give the interpretation [….] so does the patient! But the patient doesn't think: *"I am now going to precipitate. I am now going to be immature".* The patient says what he thinks. Why not? It's much easier for the analyst to draw his attention to what he thinks. I could say about this, I might say:

You are feeling that I don't know much about the real world. I don't know much about people, so there is the feeling that I do not know how grown up you are, what an awful lot of human beings know, who come to me. What am I doing that shows that I misjudge you, or anybody else, so badly? How have you discovered that I am a very bad analyst? That I don't know much about this, that I am a very bad analyst, who thinks that a baby is just a baby.

P1:   Could another patient [….]

P2:   Or he behaved *"my whole"*,[1] his whole life was the father. Does this precipitate the laws of the Universe and he acts like he was a God?

Bion: Well, you could ask him. You could say that you think he is behaving in such way and you could say:

I am quite well aware that you think lots of other things as well, but I'm drawing attention to the fact that you think, what you've just said and you can compare that with these other ideas that you've got.

The advantage of bringing out these feelings here is not that they are right or wrong, but that you can compare them with other ideas of yours. That when I say: you think that I am a very bad analyst, you can compare that with other sources you have got, when you have come here this morning. Because, if I was right and if you were right in thinking that I am a very bad analyst, then there is a problem; how did you get here this morning?

P: How did you?

Bion: Get here. How did you come to be in the consulting room. Yes and how did the bad analyst come to be in a consulting room, either? If the analyst knows so little about human beings, how does he manage to get, what miracle has he done which has enabled him to have an office, a consulting room of his own and even to get a patient to come to him. So, either it's not true, it's not the only idea that he's got – the idea that you know – the state of a baby and so on… is telling you something that isn't true. He doesn't really believe that you are thinking he's only a baby, then why is he saying so? Or if he is saying so, how does he manage to come and stay in the same room as yourself, at the same time?

A: I don't know because [….] the patient … he doesn't [….]

Bion: Try saying to him this:

I wasn't there, so I don't know what she did and I've no doubt that what you are saying is right, but as well as what you say, as well as the ordinary meaning of it, which I'm not bothering you about, because you know what it means better than I do, but as well as that you are saying this to me, because it's the only way in which you can say: 'tell me something, which you couldn't tell me in ordinary language'.

In short, I think as well as what you've already told me, not instead of, but as well as, what you've already told me, you're also feeling that I am a very bad mother. But I am a mother that does miracles. I am a mother who needs miracles to bring you up, as well as that, I think it is your way of telling me that you feel, that I'm not your mother at all. I am the wrong thing. If you set out towards me, you know I'm not even your blood relation; indeed, there is a feeling that I'm both: a bad mother, who doesn't work by miracles and I'm also the good, but psychoanalytic or black, mother. In other words, you're coming to your mother, although you know that I'm not even the right sex and in this way, you are behaving as if I am only an analyst, who was better when you're a very important miraculous mother. But, this mother is a very important one. It is one who doesn't do sexual things and who then expects the baby to be brought up, I don't know how, by miracle.

A: By miracle.

Bion: Yes.

A: He [….]

Bion: Then, I would point out that he too isn't indebted to anybody. But, as far as I, the analyst, is concerned, the wonderful thing isn't that, he is still not cured, but that he still manages to exist, in spite of the fact that I don't put him through the birth. I don't come home with him and look after him. Indeed, I only talk. If he comes next time, he thinks again that I'll only probably talk. The wonder really is, as he feels, that he's got here again, isn't dead, that we told him so. But, there's also this fact, that the analyst has got there too. So, nobody has killed him so far. So, there are two people there, neither of whom have been killed, so far.

P: [....]

Bion: Well, I'd say that there are two guilty people. There's the murderer and there's the murdered person, who hasn't died yet. There are both of them not obeying the rules.

P: Yes [....]

Bion: That part of his reason for coming is a bit clearer, because he is afraid that he has enough common sense to know that he, himself, is not a baby any more. Now, as a baby, however murderess or hostile he could be, he wouldn't be able to kill the mother and the mother could stop him, but nobody could be any sort of a mother, unless it was a miraculous mother, who could stop him to die. So, I could say:

You are afraid that you still would like to murder this person, only you can not feel that you are too feeble to murder anybody. Now, what you are anxious about is: if you allowed yourself to change, instead of coming to me for analysis and going back to childhood and all that again, something happened that made you able to realize that you are grown up.

Now, the first person who is liable to get murdered would be either the analyst or himself. So, he's very frightened of any change, because a change would make it possible now for him to do what he couldn't do, as mentioned to a child.

We'll have to stop because it's time, you see.

P: Yes.

Note

1 Transcriber's Note: Although it seems incomprehensible, that was what was said.

Supervision D6 commentary

José Renato Avzaradel

Commenting on a supervision conducted by Bion is an exciting and difficult challenge. Feeling a little uneasy, I started asking myself if I would be able to handle this mission. The unease increased after reading the supervision. When I asked myself why, I remembered a type of text in which only the speech of one of the participants in the dialogue was written. And that is what I did. Below I will group all the lines of the analyst – and the translator, which will enable a more precise idea of the material submitted to Bion's supervision.

Analyst:

– He is forty-eight years old and had already been in analysis twice. He had ten years of experience with analysis before looking for Dr. X. He has undergone analysis with him for two and a half years. He is a patient coming from a Brazilian, as they say, "noble family" ancestry.

Translator"

– Ancestors.
– He was apparently rich, but now he is very poor.
– Yes, he told me.
– I do not remember.
– Yes, he said that.
– I do not remember!
– Yes, I understand.
– He wants a miracle…
– And when I do…
– May I ask you a question?
– Always the same?
– And speaking as if it actually was, but this makes me […].
– You can do it […].
– Which means that I can […].
– Now I understand why this patient sometimes accuses me […]
– Is the analyst wrong?

DOI: 10.4324/9781003439233-13

- I do not know why [....] the patient... He does not [....]
- By some miracle.
- He [....]

This way of ordering the clinical material exposes the scarcity of information. There are practically no data on the patient: the reasons why he has searched for analysis, his personality features, how the sessions are conducted, some interpretation, the impression made on the analyst, etc. At times, the analyst even said that he did not remember what had happened. The only relevant data is that the patient wanted a miracle. Evidently, the lack of information creates a significant degree of difficulty in supervising and in commenting the supervision.

I wondered about the brackets, their possibilities, but I can only count on what I have, as Bion wrote: "There is an inexhaustible background of ignorance on which to base ourselves- and this is all we have to base ourselves on". It is often with this background of ignorance that we face in analytical work, which requires the analyst to be able to withstand not understanding until some pattern emerges.

At the beginning of the supervision, given the lack of clinical material, Bion invites the analyst to speak about the patient's expectations regarding the analysis. These expectations, Bion tells us, will always be present in all analyses, even before the first contact, and become an essential point to be examined: what actually fosters in this patient the desire to be analyzed? What does he expect? To become someone else? To be able to hear what he has never heard, assuming that the analyst has this knowledge?

Bion's questions do not seem to aim at only seeking answers, but also, and mainly, to expand the psychoanalytic field, to elicit associations. Here we see Bion stressing an essential issue, but, in addition, also inviting the analyst to say more, to bring more materials, assuming he has them. However, all he reaps is: "I don't remember" or "I understand". It is possible, then, that the psychoanalyst may say more: "He wants a miracle". – This is an impacting speech, because it makes clear that the analyst also wants a miracle: that Bion could supervise a session without sufficient elements. The intent is not to achieve the goals of human beings, but to obtain miracles. What Bion emphasizes is that there is an expectation of a God who does not have to be restricted by the laws of nature. This is a quite common fantasy. And it is difficult to give up the desire for a miracle, the eagerness to find a God. The issue of yearning for a miracle permeates the entire supervision.

Still on page three, Bion recalls that not only in the interviews, but all the time, one must examine what the patient is expecting from the analyst and, in the case at hand, what the analyst expects from Bion. Will he be God? At this point it seems that, due to the absence of material to be supervised, Bion begins to show the analyst how he can work. "You may say this or that, but to say this or that you must have some evidence to support what you say, otherwise the patient will continue to want you to be God". What is implicit is that the analyst wants Bion to be God, hence the question that emerges and imposes itself: "In short, who is the God of God?".

At this point, Bion offers his mind to the analyst to help him to think, and suggests several hypotheses, with the likely intention of provoking associations. "Does the patient want more analysis?" Does he want explanations? Why did he return? Bion seems to try to bring the situation of the clinical setting to the supervision situation. What makes it possible for the patient and the analyst to be in the same consultation office? So, there must be something other than a miracle. Bion follows an idea that seems to me of the utmost importance when he says: "Suppose this is the session"; try to bring the emotional atmosphere of the session to the supervision. But wouldn't he also be suggesting that some of the issues being worked on in the supervision would be more adequately addressed in the analyst's analysis? This is an experience, I believe, that all analysts who have conducted supervisions clearly identify and that all psychoanalysts have already experienced in their supervision.

At this point of the supervision, Bion refers to a concept which he explores in various texts and, particularly, in "Attention and Interpretation" and "Transformations" among others, which is the concept of *vertex*. A variable that he claims to mean nothing, but that points to source. From where, from what place is the fact being observed? For example, the vertex of those who undergo applied psychoanalysis is different from the vertex of the psychoanalyst, the vertex of medicine is necessarily different, and thus he concludes: differences in theories are symptoms of vertex differences, not a measure of difference. With the concept of *vertex*, theories will have the usefulness that they cannot have with another concept. Next, Bion points to a concept he called *constancy*. That is, as much as a patient may change, he will remain the same person. Aspects of his personality will remain identical; the patient remains the same. Here it is worth mentioning what Bion developed under the name of the *theory of invariance*, that which will always be the same. Transformation implies invariance, that is, so that an experience is transformed, some elements of the source situation cannot vary, they must remain invariant, otherwise it would not be a transformation, but another situation.

Bion then begins to elaborate a systematic analysis of interpretations, the way they should be built. Both what could be said to the patient, and in what language it should be said and how it should be said. In the translation into Portuguese of "Cogitations", Esther and Paulo Sandler wrote about the care and precision in the use of language that Bion always sought when communicating his ideas, and which we find in his texts and also in his supervisions.

Giuseppe Civitarese wrote in his work "Bion's Evidence and – his – Theoretical -Style" that "he develops a personal vocabulary that reflects the analyst's subjectivity. It is not just a matter of choosing effective words, or formulating effective expressions, but forging his personal style". And Bion (1976, 21) wrote about this in "Evidence":

I think that each analyst has to go through the discipline – which cannot be provided for him by any training course that I know – of forging his own language and keeping the words that he uses in good working order. ... but it is very important that it should be the one that he chooses for himself. Nobody can tell you how you are to live your life, or how you are to think, or what language you are to speak. Therefore, it is absolutely essential that the individual analyst should forge for himself the language which he knows, which he knows how to use, and the value of which he knows – knows so well that he can detect, when he gives an interpretation and the analysand repeats it with a slight change of intonation of emphasis, that although it sounds as if it is a repetition in fact it is not.

In the introduction to the book *Melanie Klein Hoje* [Melanie Klein Today], Elizabeth Spillius recalls that, for Bion, the analyst's speech must be in tune with his personality. It must have his own style; it cannot be stereotyped. Here we notice how Bion begins to scrutinize how to make an interpretation. The analyst's speech must sound real, so that it can truly be received by the patient. For Bion, when making an interpretation, one must always seek the immediate emotional reality of the analytical experience.

Bion then continues to discuss interpretations, but seen from a different vertex. When speaking about what parents could tell children about sex, Bion stresses that the information conveyed to the child must be understandable. The child must not be left unanswered, but information must be conveyed in a way that the child can understand. Likewise, the analyst must make an interpretation in such a way that it is understandable to the patient. He cannot be evasive, as the patient will respond to the issue in some other way. Nevertheless, if the interpretation is not understandable, it will become an imposition. At this point in the session, the analyst seems to have his first insight and says: "Now I understand why this patient is accusing me". Bion then makes a significant observation: that certain situations should be seen in analysis, and that the supervisory situation does not enable them to be worked on properly. Then, he adds further propositions related to interpretations.

As Bion goes on, he repeatedly stresses the concept of *evidence*. In order to make an interpretation, it is essential to examine what evidence the patient is offering us to support that understanding with. What evidence did the analyst see or think he saw?

He warns us about not getting into some kind of argument, like I am right, and you are wrong. This would be endless, useless, and even harmful. He suggests that 'feelings' are useful not because they are correct, but because they enable associations and, consequently, a mental expansion. And he ends this exposition on how one should interpret by making a thought-provoking statement: interpretations are not just words, but constructions. The impression we have is that, given the precariousness of the clinical material presented, even without any interpretations by the analyst, Bion provides us – apparently without intending to do so – with a lesson on how one should interpret.

On the subject of how to build an interpretation, let us briefly return to Freud, who considered the need to relieve the analyst's defense from his sadistic impulses. To do this, one must hold their anxiety. The analyst's duty is to help the patient recover himself. What is sought in psychoanalysis is a greater level of integration – neither a cure nor a miracle.

All of these aspects are highlighted by Bion in this supervision. Referring to Freud's *Constructions in Analysis*, Bion reflects on how interpretations not just unveil the repressed unconscious, but build new contents, actual paramnesias. In relation to these, he references Freud: "As Freud put it, individuals suffer from amnesia and create paramnesias to fill the voids. It would be great if only the patients did that and just as fortunate if we did not". As Bion asserted (1976, 22), in his work on evidence:

> and if we were feeling at all tired and more than usually ignorant, it is useful to reach out for the nearest paramnesia that is handy, the nearest psychoanalytic theory that you find lying about. Would it not be awful if the whole of psychoanalysis turned out to be one vast elaboration of paramnesia, something intended to fill the gap – the gap of our frightful ignorance?

Bion warns us there is the risk that in difficult situations we may resort to paramnesia or perhaps to some psychoanalytic theory in order to calm us down.

Bion then returns to the topic of miracles, saying: "Someone is expecting a miracle". He points to an emotional turmoil; not only the patient's, but also to something that involves the analyst (we will always be wrong), which generates anguish that is carried over to the supervision session: "Suppose this is the session". Nevertheless, now he introduces a new and disturbing element: "Well, I would say that there are two people at fault, there is the murderer and the one murdered, who has not died yet. There's both of them not obeying the rules, so nobody has killed him until now". Unless there was a miraculous mother who could keep him from dying. The issue of life and death takes shape.

This matter and the number of times Bion referred to the concept of evidence, led me to look for his work "Evidence", and what had been written about it. This text, written three years before he died, has a striking feature. Bion rarely published his own clinical materials; however, in this work he does so and with unusual courage, by presenting analytical material on a patient who killed himself. The idea of death is present at the end of this supervision in an impacting way. Giuseppe Civitarese (2013) says with intense poetic expressiveness about this honest and touching moment in which Bion exposes himself:

> "Evidence" (1976) is pervaded by a tone of bitter and skeptical wisdom. It is grief work. What Bion expresses in this text is sarcasm and pity toward himself, and pain and fury toward a patient who committed suicide. It is atonement in the sense of unison/ identification (at-one-ment) and expiation, a coming together of anger and despair. "Evidence" is a painful meditation on a dramatic personal and professional failure, which, due to the extraordinary fascination of the text, is transformed — as in Philip Roth's novels — into a sense of awe at the beauty of human existence and indignation at the horror that all this must end. … "Evidence" is something that is there but cannot be seen; it is the evidence of a person's death, the evidence of death.
>
> (p. 630)

Thus, Bion uses the scarcity of material to raise issues that permeate all analyses and all human beings. He seeks to bring to the supervision the mental environment that seems to him to be that of the analysis. And finally, he tries to show us how, and based on what, one should structure an interpretation.

In this supervision, Bion seems to seek to abstract general truths from the particulars of the supervision material and this is a classic psychoanalytic attitude. One aspect pointed out, and which is present in all analyses, is how much the patient expects from the analyst. That the analyst shows him what he still does not know and, in particular, the reason that brings him to treatment. It is a transference issue that starts even before the first interview. Being able to say what the patient does not know, seems obvious, but it is quite common for us to say things that the patients already know. This is not what they are there for.

Bion adds the idea that we must look for evidence behind some kind of lie. Let me add that, often behind some kind of truth, an even deeper truth lurks. As Civitarese recalls, we must not forget that the concepts of evidence and truth are difficult to differentiate. Based on the proposition of evidence, Bion highlights some of the peculiarities of the psychoanalyst's practice:

> There is a world in which it is impossible to see what the psychoanalyst can see… we see certain things which the rest of the world does not see… We may be dealing with things which are so slight as to be virtually imperceptible, but which are so real that they could destroy us almost without our being aware of it. That is the kind of area into which we have to penetrate.

This supervision conducted by Bion goes beyond being merely a technical class. It places us in touch with the issue of life and death being present in, perhaps, all the patients we treat, as well as in ourselves and that, precisely for this reason, we often do not realize it. The perception of this mental reality redefines our responsibilities and commitments as psychoanalysts. If this points to deeper waters, it repositions us in a different perspective. The 'harsh' use of any theoretical body, as well as the search for a miracle or even a cure, sound to me as a defense by the psychoanalyst himself so as to not be surprised by anxieties in the order of life or death. Thus, we seek protective certainties in the face of the unexpected. But shouldn't it be our job to make room for the unexpected?

References

Bion, W. 1965. *Transformations*. London: Marshfield Library.

Bion, W. 1970. *Attention and Interpretation*. London: Tavistock Publications.

Bion, W. 1976. Evidence. In *Clinical Seminars and other works*. London: Karnac, 2008, p. 312–320.

Bion, W. 1992. *Cogitations*. London: Karnac. [(2000) *Cogitações*. Rio de Janeiro: Imago, translated by Ester Sandler and Paulo Cesar Sandler].

Civitarese, G. 2013. Bion's "Evidence" and his Theoretical Style. *The Psychoanalytic Quarterly*, Volume LXXXII, Number 3, pp. 615–633.

Freud, S. 1937. Constructions in Psychoanalysis. *SE*. Vol. XXIII, pp. 255–270.

Spillius, E. 1988. *Melanie Klein Today*. Vol. 1. London: Routledge. [(1991) *Melanie Klein Hoje*. Rio de Janeiro: Imago].

Spillius, E. 1988. *Melanie Klein Today*. Vol. 2. London: Routledge. [(1990) *Melanie Klein Hoje*. Rio de Janeiro: Imago].

Chapter 7

Supervision D1

A: This patient that has been with me for... this is the one that was first with an analyst who died.

Bion: Was first?

A: An analyst that died. She was all the time biting[1] me and she used to speak more about her family: mother, father, brothers and dogs – very [little] about her husband and sons.

Bion: She was married and had what?

A: Three sons.

Bion: Three sons, yes!

A: The eldest one she doesn't like him very much. It's not that she doesn't like him, she's a little afraid of him – he's no good. But, the second is the one that she likes. The third one is in the middle!

When she arrived, she looked at me, but at the same time, I have the impression that she is away.

Bion: Yes.

A: During this session, she has this: she speaks and stops. This thing that I said...

[here Dr. Bion says something, a short phrase, but which, due to the sound, we cannot understand]

...it looks like an organic thing. This week, Monday, I think, she spoke about her sons. They looked, in the beginning, as if they were not surprised and very sad, because the dog died. But, during the weekend, they showed that really they were deeply shocked by that, because, one was very, very nervous, very anxious, all the weekend.

Bion: Yes, yes.

A: The other one is the little one. The second one had to buy a tay [tay or tie?] for himself and the older one, I don't know, but has some trouble also.

She said that they were deeply shocked by the death of the dog. Then, they went to a beach, near x and she was looking at the people surfing and they said how beautiful surf is! How it is something that you can show all your body! Your life and have some realization... And something like...

Bion: Physical expressions.

DOI: 10.4324/9781003439233-14

A: Even physical expression, but she said also, in another sense, that in a play, people are not fighting together. They are not in the way of one another. It is not like tennis, chess, etc... there is no competition.

Bion: Yes.

A: I remember that I made some observation that they need some support and she said: *"No, no, this is [not true] at all because, if you say like that, then the tennis also needs some... [racket]..."* I don't know what...

Bion: The racket!

A: The racket and the football match needed the ball...

Bion: Yes.

A: And all games are the same, but, surf has no competition.

Bion: What brothers and sisters has she got?

A: She has four brothers and one sister. She is the youngest, she said that she was very spoiled by the others.

Bion: Yes, but no children after her?

A: No children after her. She says that she has two psychotic brothers, one sister and one brother. The one that frightened the mother, that perhaps she will be killed.

Bion: Humhum.

   [The impression one has here at this point, is that this last fact had been previously mentioned to Dr. Bion].

A: You said about what brothers they are, all were linked with competition. My patient's is a psychologist and she knows I have many doctors, she knows they are having training which she can't...

Bion: She can't because...?

A: In X there is no psychologist, no society. Even I don't know if it's because of that, because, she can go to XX, if she wants to.

Bion: She's wanting to get...

A: She never said that she would like to; very few times she said that she would like to – but not really interested, she is working without it.

Bion: But, you didn't get the impression that she felt really very much about it?

A: About it no, but, about the jealousy of the others, yes!

Bion: Yes.

A: Related more with myself, I think; for [example]: I send patients to the others and not to her, something like that.

Bion: Does she think that you can't send them to her, or that you don't want to?

A: She never said directly: *"You don't send me"*, she never said: *"You send to the others, you don't send to me"*.

Bion: What was your impression about this? Did you feel she notices the fact that you don't send her any?

A: When she knows that somebody, that is my patient, has some patient that she knows, she says about this: *"I have a cousin that is with your patient"*, then, behind, is a link of jealousy.

Bion: Yes.

A: But she never said directly. Then, she spoke again about the surf all the week. She said that her youngest son said about the people that are doing the surf, that they look – is a slang, slang expression *"fera"* – *"Fera"*, is wild beast.[?feral]

Bion: Hum, Yes.

A: I pointed to her that this word... what she was trying to show me as so beautiful – the wild beast – was exactly what she has been doing with me; even on Monday, when she said *"You are no good"*. She thinks that the good, the beautiful, the marvelous, is to be a wild beast.

Bion: Yes.

A: She was furious against me, she said that it was true that she was [biting] me, that I'm no good. But, it was her son that said, that they are wild beasts.

Bion: Yes, did you point out to her, that she was making use of what her son said, to talk to you? Because, people very often say: *"Arh! yes, but I didn't say that, my son, or somebody else said it"*.

A: Yes, it was what she said.

Bion: What I usually say about that is:

> *Yes, I know that but, you are using what your son said as a way of talking to me. You're using your son's method of expressing his ideas about this, in order to express something to me, which you wouldn't be able to express otherwise. If there's no son there, you'll have to find somebody else to give you the idea how to describe the situation.*

I think what she is feeling that there's something that she wants to tell you, but, is finding it very difficult unless she uses the words and so on... which were used by somebody else. Because, it is, I think, you're right, this is quite a striking phrase that she uses. It seems to suggest, this kind of athletic thing, isn't peculiar to the surf riding, tennis anything, it's really felt to be something which is quite primitive, like wild animals, not civilized ones.

A: She also said: *"This is a way of speaking, you are taking the word, but the word is an expression in order to say that it is good"* and I say that: *"But, still there is some reason that this word was used"*.

         But the funny thing is that happened, I think, Monday and yesterday she brought, that the youngest son was at the table having dinner or lunch and he said: *"I don't want this food, I don't like this food"*.

         [As someone had not understood what the analyst had said she repeats it here]

         He was having lunch or dinner and then he said: "I don't like this food and I don't want this macaroni" the mother said: "If you want, you can have an egg, but you can't have spaghetti, [macaroni]".

Bion: But you can't have?

A: Spaghetti, [macaroni].

Bion: Oh!

A: Then, the son took his plate and threw it away. The mother said to him: *"Look, now you have to go away; go to your room"*. Then, she said that she went there and spoke with him: *"This is no good, what you did"*. Then, she realized what I had said. What I had pointed to her about this wild beast; that has some meaning. Then, she said: *"You are right, because, really, my son was a wild beast"*.

Bion: It's curious how it comes out. First of all, it seems to be just talking about surf riding and so forth… but in fact, the thing that she takes some time to tell her analyst is: how disturbed she is at this very primitive behavior, on the part of the sons. But, their kind of rivalry and envy and so forth… is really felt to be something nearer to that of an uncivilized person or animal than a civilized animal. So, I think that is the point that it has got, in what she is really frightened of. But, when she mentions this food, one wonders what has happened at breast – this is the youngest one?

A: The son? Yes, the youngest.

Bion: One wonders what has happened in the breastfeeding that she has done.

A: Her breast or the sons?

Bion: When she was the breast and had to feed the child, because sometimes mothers get very frightened and very upset at the extraordinary way in which a baby will behave… It's so wild and unrestrained… However, we'd better leave that alone at the moment, but I think that this is coming very near to something very primitive.

A: Yes. Do you remember that last week, you asked, many times, why this patient was coming to me.

Bion: Um hum.

A: It's not an answer, but one thing I am thinking is that she knows me since some years ago, when I did the seminars about *"Baby Observation"*.

Bion: Yes, yes! This question as to why she comes to you is not simply a question of the first session; it crops up over and over again. Next time, you can ask yourself again: why today? Why has she come again, today? It's probably something…

          [here it's impossible to make out the word].

          …it's probably because she thinks you would know what to say, or to do either: about this wild beast behavior in the son, or her own behavior, like a wild beast; but, one needn't bother about that very much, the really important thing is: the patient comes to you because she has some…

A: Something to say?

Bion: Hope you see, that you will know how to deal with it. It's very important to realize that, because we get so used to experiencing hostility and so forth… that patients, that we, are liable to forget that, nevertheless, patients come and they come for assistance, because they believe that they can get it. But, one forgets the positive side of it, so you need to remember that she does in fact come. Is she fairly regular, or…?

A: Yes, fairly regular, but, as I said, most of the time telling that she doesn't like me – she only comes because there is nobody else to come to.

Bion: Yes, yes.

A: And all this stuff. She only missed, I think, three sessions.

Bion: That statement can also be a statement of her idea of that's why you come. That you only see her because you've got nothing else to do and so on… not because you're interested in her or her family, that's her fear. So, the point about this is patients very often think: well, it's natural for you to see them, it's your profession and you earn a living that way and you're a psychologist or a psychoanalyst and she probably gets this idea from psychologists. So, she can be afraid that if you spoke the truth about it, you'd have to admit you don't really want to see her, at all.

      So that, in this matter, it's very difficult to come to you and tell you what her troubles are as if you were a friend of hers, as if you were friendly disposed. She hopes that you are, that's how she's got there so far. But, I think that if you can, you should draw her attention to the fact that she is afraid that as well as her not wanting to come and so forth… one is not saying that she wants to come, she's afraid that you don't want to come either; whether you are felt to be a sort of a mother, or husband, or wife there's still the anxiety that she might want to come to you, but you mightn't want to see her.

A: Yes and when her…

       [one word which is impossible to make out]

       …is on the top, the high, even attacking, she has some little words that are like that: *"But I will stay with you, I will come again".*

Bion: Um hmm.

A: Like if she has to come: *"I hope you will still be here".*

Bion: Yes, it's difficult for the patient to say that because, it's dangerous, because you might say: *"No, I'm not going to see you".*

A: Yes, I think she's afraid sometimes.

Bion: Yes, yes! So, I think you have to draw her attention to this point, if possible, without making her afraid, that you secretly don't want to see her.

A: It is my feeling, really, I don't feel that I will not like to see her. I feel sometimes near despair really, when the attack is so… I ask what can I do? What she really… what can I say? Because when she says: *"You are no good"*, always the same words, the same thing, *"I don't know what I am doing here"*, sometimes I am…

Bion: What do you think that you are? Who is this, or what is this that she's attacking like that? Because, I think that we ought, all of us, to consider what is this attack about? On the face of it, if it's made against the analyst and so on… we needn't trouble about that very much, but what is she attacking?

A: She is always comparing: *"My first analyst was too strong"*. He was very strong and she liked him very much. Her father also is a very strong man, he's dying, but as a...

[a latecomer says: *"Excuse me, good afternoon, I'm so sorry!"*]

Bion: Good afternoon.

A: The father is very rich, is a powerful man and the last analyst also... I am the feeble... I don't [push her, I don't push her] to her father. I had the impression that if she can attack me, feel me feeble, I am alive if I become strong, then I will die also.

Bion: One has to think of it in terms, again, that it sounds very primitive. It sounds as if it really is on that kind of breast feeding level, this wild animal and so forth... Now, a baby, I think, doesn't really make much difference between a father and a mother – not at first. So that, the baby expects to be put to the breast whether it's by the father or the mother. So, when it begins to find that the father does not behave like the mother, presses out toward this object and instead of finding it, getting a breast, it gets something else. So, I think that in this respect, probably, you are much more the person who does not put her to the breast. All that you do is: just talk. It's difficult to say, because, that's what everybody expects, analysis is only talk; nevertheless, if she is expecting to get something good, such as an infant might experience if it were put to the breast, then, it is a very great shock.

A: Because she's afraid of [biting]?

Bion: Afraid of you.

A: Afraid of me.

Bion: Of being a sort of dying, hostile mother, a bad mother. A mother who doesn't put her to the breast. But, that is another way of saying the father, I think.

A: The father is between?

Bion: The father doesn't put babies to the breast.

A: Then, there is no danger!

Bion: Well she is afraid of danger. What is this stranger, that doesn't put her to the breast?

A: Today she compared her mother with another wife. She is always complaining about her mother, in the way that the mother is feeble, for instance, today she said that the mother was very tired. Yesterday, her mother arrived in her room and she was lying in the side, like that.

[the position was probably shown here].

Bion: Yes.

A: Then the mother said: *"You are so tired, why are you like that? You have to turn around, this is better for a rest"*. She said: *"My mother is like that. If I go there and I sit down in a chair, she says: 'Why are you in this chair reading a book? Why are you not there?'"*

Bion: Yes.

A: *"She's kind, she wants to help me, but she doesn't do the things, she doesn't help really"*. The other is a kind of servant – is higher than servant – [governess] in the house, a woman that helps her very much in the house, while she is working. *"This woman is different, she knows I will do this..., I will do that..."*, always with something that she likes, she helps, she buys things for the house, she directs the other servants what they have to do, she pays her bills, many things. She was comparing both behaviors: the behavior of the mother and the other woman. Then, her idea about her mother is of a poor mother, [unintelligent],[has feelings but even feelings she thinks that are not directly]. She is afraid of somebody getting ill, etc. She's very critical about her mother. Really, I think she is very critical of everybody, even more about her mother, her husband and the eldest son.

Bion: See, one feels, she must be comparing it with somebody all these people who are not very good, must be in comparison with somebody who is good. So, perhaps, later it will get a little bit clearer about who this is that's so good.

A: In the moment, it's the father, the analyst who died, even herself, because she is comparing her behavior with her husband's behavior, for instance, she said: *"My husband is now beginning to drink"*. I asked something about what she was saying about this: to drink and she said: *"Oh, always before the dinner he takes a whisky. This weekend he had a whisky after beer, then he went to bed, he slept and this was the weekend..."*

Bion: In a way, it's as if she felt she's always expected to do better than her father, better than her mother, but when she's in the position of being a parent herself, she finds it's not so easy, she finds that the mother, since she is one of them, really has quite a job.

A: The husband, she can't speak with.

Bion: And the children.

A: The children.

Bion: But, all that, she expects to be easy. Yes, it is something that I have to show to her. Perhaps now, she can see that is not easy to cope with.

Bion: Well, that is what she is finding out, but she didn't like finding it out. She would like to feel that she could prove how much better she brings up her family and her husband and sons and so forth... than her father and mother brought her up. But, in fact, it's not coming out that way.

A: She says that the husband is not able to speak with the sons, because he works, he sleeps, he drinks. She compared him to herself and she says: *"I went with my sons to the beach. I spoke with the youngest one, showing to him the wild beast"*. But, when I pointed to her: *"Look, three days ago, you were furious with me because I talked about the wild beast"*.

Bion: Do you know anything about her husband?

A: About her husband? If I know? Only the things that she says.

Bion: Yes, you don't know other information at all?

A: Yes, because he is a doctor that I know about – he's a gynecologist.

Bion: So you know about.

A: But I don't know him. Yes, I know about him.

Bion: Yes, yes.

A: I know that...

Bion: Does she expect you to know about him or does she think that you know about him?

A: Yes, she knows that I know that he is a gynecologist, and very well.

Bion: Yes.

A: But, she knows that I never saw him. This is a characteristic of her: when I say something she protests. Sometimes three or four days later she say something... she says the same that I had said, but if I say again, she still will not accept it.

Bion: Yes, It is right when she says it, wrong when you say it. So, it's a part of the rivalry situation in which it's impossible for you to be right. If the interpretation is the right interpretation, then, it's her idea. Very tiring to deal with patients like that, because you get no knowledge of any of the work you do.

A: In the moment, yes, but three or four days later, I can realize that she, at least, heard what I said.

Bion: Yes, but three or four days later she hasn't acknowledged that you said it.

A: Yes.

Bion: Doesn't matter very much perhaps, although, I think that it does matter this way that the patient is not really showing any capacity for affection or appreciation. She may be capable of affection or appreciation, but she's not showing it. Well now, the trouble with this is this: one doesn't want patients to show affection or appreciation particularly, but it is as if the patient does not somehow get around to developing their side, that part of their personality. That is the danger with a baby like this, who behaves in that wild beast fashion. You can't let him do it, because he will go on like that and then, he won't learn anything better, till it's far too late. If this patient doesn't learn to expect, or to express feelings of appreciation with you, very doubtful where she will have a chance to learn how to do it.

A: She only, in the first and second week of the treatment, she was happy with me and said that she liked the way I was working and she looked as if it was right. I told you, she had a dream that I interpreted, about something sexual with me.

Bion: That she was doing something sexual in company with you.

A: Not doing, but, wanting... I remember, because it had some sexual link.

Bion: Yes.

A: During the session, I didn't notice any reaction really, but the next day she said she was feeling happy, because she talked that she could say anything she wants.

Bion: How did she know it was you?

A: How did she know?

Bion: How did she know it was you in the dream?

A: I don't know, I said. I linked some.

Bion: Who did she say it was in the dream?

A: I don't remember the dream, but there is – something in a park, something like that, because, the next day she said: *"Now, I know that I can be with you in a bench in a park, a square and talk with you and feel I am alone, even if there are a lot of people around".*

Bion: Yes. Now, that point, one would like to know how does she know that? Because, after all, analysands talk about analysts. They're always discussing their analysts and so forth... Why do they think that their analysts don't talk about their patients to other analysts? Now, what has made her think that you wouldn't do that? The point is this: one doesn't want to give the impression that one does, so I think that I'd like to say something as though: *"Well, I am not trying to tell you that I do talk to other people about your private affairs, but I would like to know why you think that I wouldn't?"* So, it's important that this patient should admit what it is about you, that makes her trust your discretion, or your loyalty to your patients. See, as she's going on, apparently, there is nothing good to be said for you, but nevertheless, she's still coming. And if you're as bad as all that, why is she still coming?

A: Yes and the trouble is: I think that what she said – that she was not afraid – was not what she was feeling. I think this, because from that moment, she changed and I began to be the bad one.

Bion: Yes.

A: Now, I think, perhaps, is the contrary that what she had said, she's afraid to be with me. She's not trusting me.

Bion: You have to think of it in this way: how often would you talk about your private affairs to a complete stranger? Yet, in analysis, that is what happens! One of the reasons one goes to an analyst is because the analyst isn't part of the social setup. Now, how do people come to trust an analyst to be discreet or even loyal? She ought to, she should at some point, say what has lead her to believe that you are trustworthy.

A: Yes, because she's still coming.

Bion: Because she's still coming and it is very extraordinary that anybody goes to a stranger and, indeed, even if anybody who isn't a stranger, who knows other people in the district and so forth... Because, as far as she knows, she's got no reason to suppose that you wouldn't talk to anybody about her. So that if she told you anything private, you might spread it all over the place. She would certainly spread anything all over the place about you.

A: And she used, she...

Bion: Then that... at anything...

       [Dr. Bion says a word which is impossible to make out]

...then, why does she think that if she can do it, that the analyst wouldn't do it?

A: Yes. One of the ways that she uses to attack me is like that. Not directly, usually she is like that: *"I went to a meeting – a psychologist meeting – then, somebody asked me: what about your analysis, are you having one?"* or something like that and she says something like: *"Oh no, she is baroque, she is old fashioned"*.

Bion: She told you this?

A: Yes, she told me this...

Bion: Yes, yes!

A: Always that she is saying this to another. If somebody asks something about me, I am awful, I am...

Bion: Now, the question is: why doesn't she think that you would be able to say the same thing, if she really believed that she wouldn't come to you? Why doesn't she really believe it? We get so used to this fact: that we are really supposed to preserve a discretion, not pass on other peoples private affairs, that one fails to recognize what a highly...

[someone coughing covers the word]

...that psychoanalysts accept. Parents don't usually talk and say anything about their children, in the way that children say things about their parents. But, this isn't children and parents, this is an analysand and analyst. Here it were just true and talking about that part of the mother as well, one wouldn't mind very much, but when it is grown-ups talking about other grown-ups, that's serious. It's extraordinary how people who are supposed to be psychiatrists and so forth... will quite freely and easily say: *"Oh, so and so, he's mad, she's mad"*. Yes, but doctors are not supposed to give diagnosis like that. There aren't any evidences, really; for a doctor to say that about another doctor is slander. Now, just because it is psychoanalysis this patient thinks she can say all these things about you, but you won't say them back about her. One doesn't want to pretend that one would, but one does want to draw attention to the fact that the patient trusts you not to do so.

Well, we've got to the time! Yes.

Note

1   Editor's Note: It is unclear if this is a direct translation of a Portuguese expression for "angrily snapping at" someone or if the patient actually bit the analyst. See the discussion that follows.

Supervision D1 commentary

Claudio Castelo Filho

My first reaction upon reading this supervision was bewilderment.[1] Apparently not only Bion but also the presenter and the participants supposed they knew what the presentation was about; it was purportedly related to a previous supervision they still remembered. The conversation sounded disjointed and bewildering – I was in doubt as to the gender of the analyst. At first it seemed to be a woman, but only later, when the Portuguese feminine article – 'a' – appeared I confirmed it was really a female analyst. Perhaps this confusion was related to an issue of undifferentiation between father and mother for babies. The next uncanny feature was the fact that the analysand bit the analyst, which seemed very out of place, as the translator's footnote suggests (later, however, I considered that the analysand was a wild beast who constantly abused the analyst, she was actually biting her all the time like a baby who bites the breast it needs so badly – or the breast that turns out to be a no-breast) (Bion, 1965, p. 54).

Was this a conversation in the beginning of the supervision, a conversation among surfers? I can only provide a ludicrous caricature of this kind of conversation, where people talk with monosyllabic slang words, apparently implying what is being said. What do they really talk about? It would seem that they understand each other and that what they say is obvious to the participants by means of contextual features that could not be expressed in writing.

I was prompted to search for the preceding supervision in order to grasp what it was about. But then I reconsidered. As in analysis itself, it would be better to continue with what I had, including my initial bewilderment, and to follow the course of the events.

So there were no surf competitions? Where did the analysand get that from? I am sure there were already surf competitions in the 1970s. And even surfers who do not compete on a professional basis do compete among themselves: who has the best performance, who surfs the best waves, who gets to surf a particular wave, who has the best surfboard, who has been more times in Hawaii or another surf hotspot, or who accomplishes the greater feats; there is also the contempt for the *paneleiros* (a slang word from my youth referring to beginners or untalented surfers).

An issue brought forward by Bion later during the supervision is outlined from the outset: the capability (or its lack) of having emotions. Initially the analysand's

DOI: 10.4324/9781003439233-15

children (Bion suggests that she uses them to speak about herself – projective identification) would be unable to have or show emotions. Nevertheless, the death of the dog – an event to which their first reaction is apparent indifference – soon is shown to have a deep impact on them. Also, the analysand apparently despises the analyst ('you're no good'): however, as the old Portuguese proverb goes, he who disparages a thing wants to buy it. The issue at hand is the pain associated to loss (or potential loss) that comes with love, attachment, appreciation for the loved one.

What is implied by 'there is no competition in surf'? Is this meant that 'surf' is a sphere of human activity where envy and rivalry do not operate'? The counterpoint is the perception that rivalry becomes a nodal point in this material as one reads it. Are we dealing with the hope that there might be a relationship, an experience where envy, rivalry, jealousy, and the categories of superior/inferior are not the prevailing features? Are we dealing with the analysand's expectations for what she seeks with and in her analyst? Someone able to deal with envy and rivalry in such a way that she does not compete for primacy and superiority? Was this her experience with the breast/mother and with her father? Were they parents exceedingly threatened by their daughter's development potential? Did she feel threatened by the potential development of her children? Was she engaged in fierce competition with her children? Is there also the fear that the 'pretty good' analyst with whom she is delighted – who can surf the (mental) waves she herself cannot – is also a wild beast (*fera*) in a frightful way?

Bion says that *'[i]t seems to suggest that this kind of athletic thing isn't peculiar to the surf, riding, tennis, anything; it's really felt to be something which is quite primitive, like wild animals, not civilized'*. On the other hand, sport is an important means to civilize the primitive and the wild. Instead of war, there is sport competition. It is also true that sport competition sometimes 'regresses' and degenerates into war both on the field or court and between opposing supporters. We must remark that *fera* (like all related terms in their origins) has a double meaning. *Fera* = very good; *fera* = primitive, violent, and potentially evil. What use one can make of the human potentialities? There is no creativity without primitivity. How to avail oneself of the wild primitivity in a creative fashion? A colleague of mine claims to have a one-volume edition of Bocage's[2] works that has two front covers. The book has two beginnings. One side of the book contains Bocage's gorgeous sonnets. The other side presents the author's 'pornographic', bawdy production. The editor points out that one thing does not exist without the other – both aspects share the same source. Two small books by Apollinaire – now part of the French literary canon – come to my mind: *Les Exploits d'un jeune Don Juan* and *Les Onze Mille Verges*, where the violence associated to boundless sexuality is so extreme that by the end of the second book the main character is reduced to a pile of mangled flesh. Another example are the works of Sade: they are not only a part of the literary canon but are placed on its summit. Bion points out that the writings of Freud may also be seen by many as the pornographic work of a degenerate mind (not to speak of Melanie Klein!). Freud, Klein, and Bion alike are not afraid of plunging into their own primeval worlds in order to avail themselves of them – either by creating psychoanalysis or developing it further. The *Iliad*, the *Odyssey*, all the great Greek tragedies, and the works of Shakespeare – all extraordinary, beautiful works – are essentially a melting-pot of violence, sexual assault, incest, torture, poisoning, betrayal, deceit, sweeping passion, desperate love, and all incarnations of human cruelty.

As far as I see it, the analysand is looking for someone who helps her to deal with and make good use of this primordial, primeval world without being destroyed by it or destroying the person she recruits to help her do so. This leads to the breast-feeding issues suggested by Bion. I think that the analysand was terribly afraid of being a wild baby who bites the breast, resulting in revenge taken by the latter or by its loss. From another point of view, she felt that the wild world where 'she is located' forces her to be a beast in order to survive.

In Bion's words: *When she was the breast and had to feed the child, because sometimes mothers get very frightened and very upset at the extraordinary way in which a baby will behave... It's so wild and unrestrained.*

It should be pointed out that Bion often turns to his own life experience, and to the analyst's, rather than to theoretical psychoanalytical references. As Bion himself said, if psychoanalysis were not similar to life, it would not be psychoanalysis. On page 8, he refers to the fear that the analyst too may not want to see or be with her, or that the she may wish to meet the analyst but the latter does not want to be with her.

He then proposes that the analyst should call her attention to this issue without suggesting that the analyst secretly wishes not to see her. In my opinion, this is relevant *if it corresponds to the analyst's true feelings*.

The analyst should take this truth into account: sometimes one simply does not want to meet someone. A question often made by Bion to the analyst and participants in other supervisions comes to my mind: would you like to receive this person? Would you like to continue to see him or her? Would you like to receive him or her today? And what about tomorrow? etc.

Some patients are really very dangerous wild beasts. I would like to quote some lines by Bion where he says:

That is the danger with a baby like this, who behaves in that wild beast fashion. You can't let him do it, because he will go on like that and then he won't learn anything better till it's far too late. If this patient doesn't learn to expect, or to express feelings of appreciation with you, very doubtful where she will have a chance to learn how to do it.

Are some people past the point of no return? Or are they naturally equipped with such a measure of envy and rivalry that these characteristics are the very stuff of their personality? – such as proposed by Bion in *Transformations* (p. 144) when he writes that someone's health, being oneself, being at one with one's nature, with one's normality, is being this envious person who cannot stand being helped (for being healthy would imply the very difficulties which the person creates and endures). If, as Bion proposes, analysis serves to present someone to himself so he may be himself (since no one can be cured of what he is by nature), analysis will stress these envy and rivalry features belonging to the person's nature. Am I willing, as an analyst, to cope with the consequences of this? I refer here to Freud's remark that analysis does not change someone's character (Freud, 1937).

There are those who think they do not need to pay the analyst's fee, and if you demand payment, then you are a monster who has no respect for their suffering. Others do not acknowledge any *responsibility* for what they do, quite on the contrary: they are convinced that you are responsible for everything they do – an extremely perilous situation. I recommend reading Bion's Conference Ten in Rio de Janeiro (Bion, 1974, p. 149–171), where he warned the analyst of the great risk of treating a young man who did not hold himself responsible for anything he did (not even the fact that he was undergoing analysis) and also a supervision he did in Buenos Aires where he realized it had been a serious mistake of his to treat someone in a similar situation.

I believe that treatment can evolve with people in which one observes an ineluctable need for reality, even if to their own disadvantage, i. e. they may hate this need and actually prefer (like so many do) avoidance and illusion, and yet something in them demands the truth. This is something inherent to them – psychoanalysis cannot create it, just as it cannot create emotional capability

In *Cogitations* (1992), Bion discusses tropisms (p. 34–35): *murder – seeking an object to murder or to be murdered; parasitism – seeking a parasite or host, creation – seeking an object to create or by which to be created.* Creation/creativity may be a means to parasitism or murder. On the other hand, if creation prevails as the stronger tendency in the individual, he may avail himself of the other two in a creative way. In the same book, Bion writes (p. 125):

(...) 7. A man may feel he lacks a capacity for love. 8. A man may lack capacity for love. 9. Similarly, He may feel He lacks a capacity for truth, either to hear it, or to seek it, or to find it, or to communicate it, or to desire it. 10. He may in fact lack such capacity. 11. The lack may be primary or secondary, and may diminish truth or love, or both. 12. **Primary lack is inborn and cannot be remedied; yet some of the consequences may be modified analytically.**

Later, in the São Paulo conferences (Bion, 1974), he was not so optimistic as in the last sentence quoted. In *Cogitations*, he also mentions the disaster lived by his colleague Millais Culpin (p. 103).

In this context, the analyst may not be the expected breast. Like a little baby, the analysand may not be able to distinguish father from mother; however, the analyst is supposed to make this distinction, realizing that he is not the analysand's mother nor the analysand is his baby. This has an impact on the analysand. The analyst should not attack or reproach the analysand for this confusion, but rather help him to make the distinction and develop the conditions to sustain it (which is also a way of helping him to live and somehow work-through the Oedipal situation). Who is this stranger who does not offer the breast? (p. 11).

If I am not this breast, there is the inevitable comparison that will place me far behind it. Can I, as an analyst, stand that? I regard this an essential condition to perform analysis. Even a mother, when she helps her child to develop, must tolerate from a certain point that she too is someone who does not offer the breast. She must become a no-breast in order to let the capability of thinking develop. When there is the expectation of an ideal mother/breast, it is the expectation and demand that the person requires of him- or herself. Since this is an unrealistic parameter, he or she is incapable of being a real father or mother and acting in a really useful manner. This is also a fundamental issue for real analysis. If the analyst is supposed to be an ideal breast/mother, which cannot happen, he or she will be unable to be the analyst, the real person capable of offering something real to his or her patients.

Like the patient who is not pleased to realize that she herself is not capable of the care and capabilities she expects from the others, the analysts who do not realize this in their practice and nurture the fantasy that being an analyst is a superhuman condition may also dislike or abhor realizing their true condition.

On the other hand, Bion says the following about the patient: *"she may be capable of affection or appreciation, but she's not showing it"*. I identify the following as the nodal point: the analysand must be capable of affection or appreciation. Analysis does not create or give rise to this. It must exist in the analysand. And for me this is the decisive issue determining whether an analysis can occur. The patient may not know or not want to demonstrate this, not want his affection to be perceived. Our job is to verify what causes this mechanism. Fear of loss? Of dependency? Of abuse by the person one is dependent of? Fear of pain? Fear of biting the coveted breast of which one depends? Fear of destroying by voracity the precious thing one is dependent of? Fear of driving the mother/analyst crazy with unbearable sentiments? etc.

Now we will address the issue of the analyst's trustworthiness and reliability. In this supervision, Bion refers to the possibility of analysis being used for indiscretion or gossip purposes:

> *(...) Why do they think that their analysts don't talk about their patients to other analysts(...) So, it's important that this patient should admit what it is about you, that makes her trust your discretion, or your loyalty to your patients. See, as she's going on, apparently, there is nothing good to be said for you, but nevertheless, she's still coming. And if you're as bad as all that, why's she still coming?*

The analyst is a common person, and his character and capacity may only be assessed through the analysand's direct experience with him. Being an analyst is not a guarantee of anything. An analyst can be a vicious, mentally limited, manipulative, and dishonest person. But also an ethical and well-intentioned person. Even the well-intentioned analyst is not free from faux pas or mistakes, and the analysand must be aware of that: he must know that he is dealing with someone real, and for this reason he is never exempt from responsibility for himself. Real trust in the analyst can only originate from experience and intuition. There are no other means.

I would like to stress that the analyst *is actually talking about the analysand with other people in her supervision.*

What were the supervision participants doing? One could say they were talking about the analysand. Her great fear. And what are we doing on this very occasion? Talking about this particular analysand or our own analysands? In a certain way, yes. That is precisely what we do!

However, what is the point of an analyst talking about his analysand with other analysts? Gossip? Slander? Intrigue? Looking for help in order to develop and better collaborate with the analysand? Learning to think something not yet thought? What are the precautions one must take?

Unfortunately, there are psychologists, psychiatrists and psychoanalysts who make derogatory comments about their analysands and their families.

Is psychoanalyst synonymous with good character? For me, it is a function someone performs, not his character. Like any activity, it may be performed by all kinds of people. Apart from the character issue, there may also be issues of deficient training or naïveté leading to disastrous use of the information shared. It is really necessary to protect the analysands from being identified. What is most important here is not the social information about the person, but his or her psychic dynamics during the session allowing insight into the personal characteristics that interest us.

The analysands should verify their analysts' ethical standards through their actual experience with them. Having fear is a reasonable and healthy reaction. This process involves using intuition and running some risks as they assess how their analysts effectively work. It makes perfect sense that an analysand is wary of his analyst and of potential misuse of what is disclosed in session. It is only from experience that one can judge whether an analyst is competent, honest, and well-meaning, or not. If his judgment is a negative one, he should be reasonable and act according to his perceptions. Or else realize that his initial judgment (for example, that the analyst is incompetent or dishonest) does not correspond to his actual perceptions. A third alternative would be remaining with this analyst he deems a cruel person and a bad professional, always assuming responsibility for the poor treatment he receives.

As mentioned above, the analyst too is not obliged to keep treating someone he feels is incapable of real appreciation and is more interested in annoying the analyst than benefitting from what he might offer – envy being the very stuff of the patient's personality (Bion, 1965, p. 144).

The analysand should be aware that both he and the analyst are free to discontinue the treatment whenever they feel like. If this freedom of choice by the analyst may initially come as an anguishing factor to the analysand, it may also represent great relief, since he knows that he is being treated because the analyst wishes so, and not because he is forced to do it by moral or technical reasons or only for the money.

On the other hand, to be aware that the analyst is a competent, well-meaning person may also cause anguish to the patient (this seems to be the case of the analysand in the supervision). Is not a common complaint that one cannot find a great love, but when this happens, the same person breaks up? Attaching to an invaluable being is a very frightening thing. Recognizing true value, especially if it is something never found before, is terrifying. This terror is a legitimate reaction. The experience of love and value brings with it the fear of suffering associated to loss and potential abuse by the loved one. It is necessary to develop the ability of coping with pain and suffering in order to experience passionate love – which for Bion is the condition where someone is nearest to being who he or she really is.[3]

Notes

1 The supervision was held in Portuguese (participants) and English (Bion), with an interpreter translating their talks more often than not. There were misunderstandings and doubts as to the terms used. The analyst's speech was much more confused in Portuguese than in English, where the initial conversation was less fragmented and disjointed. The double meaning of the English word, *racket*, pointed out by Bion, for example, was not noticed by the Brazilian participants or the interpreter. This double meaning does not exist in Portuguese. The word *fera*, adequately translated as *wild beast*, **does** have a **second meaning** in Portuguese: that of someone who is very competent in what he does.
2 One of the greatest Portuguese poets.
3 Passionate love' is the nearest I can get to a verbal transformation which represents the thing in itself, the ultimate reality, the 'O...' ' (Bion, 1991, p. 183).

References

Apollinaire, G. (1911). *Les Exploits d'un jeune Don Juan*. Paris: Ed. J'ai Lu, 1977.

Apollinaire, G. (1907). *Les Onze Mille Verges*. Paris: EJL, 2006.

Bion, W.R. (1965). Transformations. In: *Seven Servants: Four works by Wilfred R. Bion*. New York: Jason Aronson, 1977.

Bion, W.R. (1974). *Brazilian Lectures*. Rio de Janeiro: Imago.

Bion, W.R. (1991). *A Memoir of the Future*. London: Karnac, 1991.

Bion, W.R. (1992). *Cogitations*. London: Karnac.

Freud, S. (1937). Analysis Terminable and Interminable. In: *S.E. XXIII*, p. 216–254. London: Hogarth, 1978.

Chapter 8

Supervision D9

A: The same patient. One day when she was speaking about the *crystal*, that she would like something in analysis like a crystal. I said something about she had edges – the crystal has edges. She protested and said: *"But I am not speaking about the edges, I am speaking about the crystal, the infinite"*. I see. Then, she showed me the teapot, where she was seeing the same thing. The next day, she spoke again about the crystal and she said that she would like that our relation would be like a crystal. She was speaking about it being white and clear, that she was feeling that she herself had a lot of edges.

Bion: But, she said something about wanting to be like a crystal or... wasn't it?

A: She said that our relation – the analysis with me – she would like to be like a crystal.

Bion: Um hmm.

A: But, in the next day white, very white, very clear, transparent. But that she was feeling that she herself, she had a lot of edges.

Bion: But, was it now the white crystal or what crystal was it?

A: It's not a diamond, it's a simple crystal. Because, when I said something about idealization, she said that she was not speaking about a diamond, because if she was speaking about a diamond, then, it would be something idealized. But, she was speaking about a simple thing, something that she likes, beautiful – she didn't say the word beautiful. But, she was speaking about something pure, but not a diamond, a simple crystal. You know we have a lot of these stones here...

Bion: Yes.

A: That are like crystal, diamonds, but are not diamonds. Then she told me a dream about her father. Her father is very ill, he's near dying and...

P1:   In reality?

A: In reality, yes! In reality, he's very ill. The father was in a state of Brazil far away, where he was born and her sister-in-law – the one that she says likes very much – was saying to her that her father had no dinner.

Bion: No...?

DOI: 10.4324/9781003439233-16

A: No dinner, nothing to eat at dinner and then she said: *"Don't be worried, I will get some dinner"*.

Bion: That's the sister-in-law?

A: Eh?

Bion: The sister-in-law said that?

A: The sister-in-law says that he had no dinner and the patient said: *"I will"*.

Bion: She, your patient said?

A: Yes. *"I will get some dinner"*.

P1:   Something for him to eat?

A: Something for him to eat, yes! This was her dream, but she didn't make a direct association. What she said was that she was thinking about her father, comparing him with the mother – that the father and the brothers, they know what they want. They have some intention when they do something. They are doing projects, for instance: to have another factory, always more money, more firms, not exactly money, but power.

Bion: Something concrete.

A: Yes, and the mother was completely different. The mother was always absent. Then, she said something about a colleague, that was doing a baby observation. She remembered that, the day before, she was telling this colleague that she was very wrong in her observation, because she had to do something therapeutic with the mother – not only to observe, that something was wrong with her, because after one year of observation, the mother was still absent.

Bion: What does she mean by that; where is the mother?

A: The mother of the baby, that the colleague was observing. Because usually we want, during the baby observation, to have the mother and the baby, but the mother... you know, they have a lot of maids and servants. Usually, the servant is with the baby and not the mother.

Bion: But, she didn't say where the mother was... the mother was just absent?

A: Absent!

Bion: Yes.

A: She was insisting that we had to do something therapeutic... *"Why these colleagues that are psychologists, why they didn't do something in order to show the mother that the baby, the child needed her? We both were in one year of analysis"*. The next day, – that was yesterday – she looked at me and she said when she was lying on the couch:

> *How nice you are today! I was thinking that you were going with colleagues to X. This is so nice; I am remembering that I when I was an adolescent, that I used to go with my colleagues to some holiday, in order to do programs with the colleagues, some excursions in other towns.*

That was in a completely different way. Then, she said about her husband...

Bion: How would you characterize that difference? Would you characterize it, at all?

A: My feeling was because I said: *"Until Tuesday"*, I showed her I was not the only analyst…

Bion: No, I was meaning in what way would you say…

A: That she was different?

Bion: Yes, because, this is the sort of thing, which is so difficult to describe.

A: Yes.

Bion: I'm asking you the question… I'm well aware that the demands on verbal expression are tremendous.

A: No, not only because what she said. She, really was looking different. In the last week, she was so thin, without make-up. But it was not the make-up; perhaps yesterday, also, she had not make-up. But, she looked different. She was, even, smiling when she entered and also the way to speak. She was really different. She had not this superiority that sometimes she looks.

Bion: Yes.

A: But, she said that *I* looked different!

Bion: Yes. I think it's simply one of these things it's worth asking you the question, because, I think, it's a question which exists; you may be able to answer it, or you may be able to answer it later on, especially if you can contrast it with this more ragged worn sort of woman, on one occasion, this is a different one. So you could if there were two sisters, you might be able to compare the two, but at least…

          [Someone coughs while Dr. Bion was speaking, blurring two or three words]

          it might be useful, if not on this occasion, on some other occasion to say what the difference is. However, I think that you make it clearer to me, perhaps you can verbalize it yourself later on… I don't know. It really, in a sense, sounds almost more human, not so much the hard edges and the lines of the crystal, that sort of thing…

A: Yes.

Bion: …as if it were some kind of stone – but really a person.

A: Yes and in the material, there has something linking this, but, just typical, the same. Because, she told me about her husband, a discussion she had with him; she wants to buy land in order to have a house – she lives in a flat. It is a very beautiful place, far away from the town, but she wants to leave. The husband was very afraid because he said: *"Look, we are having another house and I am preparing my consulting room, a new consulting room and then, it is very difficult"*. She was telling me how he is afraid! Different from her father and her brothers – they are always wanting more and more. But the husband, he's afraid about money. He's afraid of not to being able to… if he buys, he cannot have the house and so on… Then, she was telling him that she would help him, because, she can sell something and then help him. But, he was still afraid. She was very sad because she wants the house.

Bion:	She wanted the house?
A:	She wanted the house. In the end she said: *"But yesterday we had a very good sexual relation – intercourse"*. Then I showed her, that she was able to speak with her husband, to dialog. Even if they were not satisfied, completely satisfied, they were able to discuss. I showed her this, as a different link. I showed her how she was speaking also differently with me, there were something different today. Yesterday it was with her husband and now with me. Then, she said that she feels that she was in a… what you call a *"cordas"*?[1] String, in a string, swinging.
Bion:	Hum…
A:	Then, she remembers the Sunday that she went in the beach with two sons and the little boy – that is the son of a servant, that the mother is keeping.
Bion:	Um hmm.
A:	And they were jumping from some stones, in the beach.
Bion:	Um hmm.
A:	And it were very difficult and then, she was near sitting…
P1:	To curve, to bend.
Bion:	Yes, yes.
A:	Bending in order to jump and this boy – the one that is not the son – came back and said to her: *"It's better if you can go straight away – not bend – if you can be walking"*.
Bion:	Um hmm.
A:	And the she tried. Jumping and really it was better. She said that she looked at this little boy and found him different from her sons. He looked so thin, not so strong as the others; but, very able to jump. Then she said that the little boy gave her his hand, in order to help her and she said she felt something so good – to have the contact of the hands. I remember that I compared the difference of being about to be in the string and to hold hands. One is an object and the other, is a human contact. She, then, told me about a picture of Michelangelo where God is near Adam with his hand.
Bion:	Um hmm.
A:	Then, she spoke more about the picture, that she likes it very much. I said to her that now she was speaking about God, was now God. And she said:

> But it's not God that I am speaking of, I am speaking about Michelangelo, who was able to do this and really, God was not touching, it's very close, but not touching the hand of Adam. I don't know what.

Bion:	Well, let's consider it a moment: does anybody get any impression… what do you suppose the emotional situation is, which she's trying to express to the analyst?
P2:	My impression is that she's trying to convey the idea of the death in her husband and…
A:	What?

P2:   Her husband and stimulate in her… she is expressing her feeling of poverty, her possibilities of helping her husband.

P2:   …

    [She utters two or three words that are incomprehensible]
    something like this?

P2:   About the lot and the house, the future.

Bion: I would have thought that, that is more than likely, but of course, if she helps her husband, it will inevitably help her. So, it's one of these actions, which is sure to be to her interest, if she is successful in doing so. Even, can one get any kind of overall picture of why this is being aroused? Why the *"so anxious"* and why *she* is so anxious, that the relationship with her analyst should be this crystalline relationship?

A: You know now.

Bion: Or… um hmm?

A: Now, I didn't think this. But, now she knew that I was coming here; then, I think, really, she was speaking about you: the God. Perhaps, there was a third person.

Bion: Yes.

A: Because, when I said *"God"*, she protested: *"I am speaking about Michelangelo"*. When she protests, it is because there is something, usually.

Bion: You could try pointing out: *"Yes, but Michelangelo is dead and one of the questions is: why are you so concerned with a dead Michelangelo?"*

P3:   But, the Michelangelo that is dead is very near the analyst.

Bion: Well, what I'm trying to do, again, is to stir something which would get this woman to say, or come a bit nearer to giving some sort of material which would explain why this discussion now.

P2:   I think that yesterday you pointed out the envy she has probably about the analyst, who was able to study and…

Bion: Yes!

P2:   Know more etc… Today, maybe, she is expressing more her fear of the analyst, who is putting so much interest in something that would put the analyst identical perhaps in this relationship. That's why I'm supposing that there is some relationship between one thing and the other. Yesterday, you said about the envy, today, maybe, she is talking about her…

    [A word is said that is incomprehensible]
    of the analyst coming here, because, to come to you is to come here – is to put herself in danger. My patient is very jealous of you, for instance, then, I could think she was very envious of me and then, I could see how much danger she would see in this 'coming to you'. There are many different feelings she's trying to pose, to show me, and maybe this is what this patient is doing.

Bion: Well, excepting that this patient has also been talking about a father who's dying.

A: And Dr. X also.

P2:   And Dr. X she has behind her all the time.

Bion: Yes, but there's also the feeling of not devoting herself to her father – a dying father.

P3:   I have the impression that she is emphasizing the fact that the analyst is well dressed, nicer and she thinks the analyst is improving in some way and she is smiling, she is gratified with hope.

Bion: The principle behind this, I think, is: the difficulty which is that, even, if the father, or mother, or husband or wife were dying, the world still goes on. If she ever, as a child, wanted to take possession of the father and be the father's wife and so on and so forth… all that could be discounted on the grounds that she couldn't be old enough, anyhow. But, not so today! Not so today, when she is a grown woman, who can have children and so on and so forth… but she does not devote herself to the dying father – who dies alone.

A: Do you think that she is guilty for that?

Bion: I think it's one of these events which helps to raise guilt to a higher pitch, especially if… as well as being alive and well, with all kinds of advantages and so on… she's also wanting to have an analysis. That's not doing anything for the husband. That seems to be rather like leaving that business to God to stretch out his hand to Michelangelo and also, to the husband who is dying and so on… But, the trouble with this is that one doesn't want to give an interpretation that sounds like saying that she ought to go and devote herself to her dying father. I think the problem is: the dying father is, in fact, too ill. All that he would like to be, would be, to be properly nursed by whoever is capable of doing it. So that, from a common sense point of view, everything would suggest that she should get on with her analysis, be successful at it and get on with her marriage and also make a success of it. But, I think that it is really felt to be very, very hard to be devoting herself, say, to her husband, or her boys, or even to getting some sort of assistance from her analyst, in a situation where she is not doing anything for the mother's husband, or for the husband's wife.

   The difficulty I see about this is: how to give such an interpretation, because, if you say something of that sort, then, it sounds to the patient, exactly as if, in your opinion, you thought that the patient should devote themselves to the parents, which isn't what one wants to say. What one wants to do is: to draw attention to the guilt there is about the fact that one does not bring up one's father or mother, one does not marry one's father, nor does one marry one's mother; but, for some reason, the universe isn't made like that. It's not made like that in the first instance and in the present, there are other things which the person concerned has to do. But what things?

   What if she is able to give her boys a nice day on the beach, an exciting companionship between the three of them and playing on the beach and so forth… that doesn't seem to be sort of grand enough, or moral enough. If she herself is really having a kind of analytical relationship, which makes her more human, that doesn't seem to be grand enough, either. So, there can be the wish to get a certain degree of support from you, to be allowed, as it were, to get on with her own life and her own affairs. Of course, if you do give support, well, you're not really being moral; but, if you don't, of course, you're really condemning her. So, it's difficult to know how to give such an interpretation. This is why it's saying: *"How would you describe the difference in feeling"*. It's not that only. It's: *"What words would you use in the course of your analysis?"* because that's the really important thing!

Once you've got your own vocabulary, it comes possible to improve it, with little bits you find and so forth… but, it seems to me, that one needs to have a basic vocabulary of one's own. I think that this is one of these difficult situations, because, the patient is really having quite an emotional experience and is in need of assistance and it puts a strain on any vocabulary. I think one might try something of this sort like:

> *You seem to be having a successful, or being able to give the children a successful day on the beach; but, you seem also to be somewhat guilty because if they have a successful day on the beach, you're bound to be that much more pleased yourself. Or, if you're able to give you husband wise advice, you seem to be a bit worried, because then, he might get that sort of house that you yourself would like to have. In short, you seem to be worried at the prospect of benefiting either: in your relationship with me, or with your family.*

P3:	I have this impression…
Bion:	Yes.
P3:	Because of the topic of the: *"swinging on the string"*; this is an idiomatic expression in Portuguese, the way the patient is talking to the analyst.
Bion:	What about that idiomatic expression?
P3:	It's a difficult position we are dancing on a swinging string. It's a difficult position.
A:	You know, when they are doing it in a circus.
Bion:	Yes, yes!
P3:	More difficult than to walk over a distended string.
Bion:	Yes.
P3:	It's difficult to…
Bion:	It's not drawn from the use of puppets, is it?
P3:	No, from the circus.
Bion:	It's more from the circus.
A:	The circus, yes! Acrobats.
Bion:	A stack wire[2]
P3:	Yes.

A: When you put your feet on and it swings.

Bion: It's more dangerous than the tight rope.

A: Yes!

P3:   More dangerous. It's difficult to express.

A: It's: *"corda bamba"*.

Bion: And the expression in Portuguese is…?

P3:   To be in a very difficult position.

A: *"Corda Bamba"*.

P3:   *"Corda Bamba!"* It's not wire, it's a tissue, but…

Bion: So you use the expression that he or she is…?

P3:   Is walking or dancing on this…

A: Swinging string.

Bion: I mean the actual Portuguese expression.

P3:   The actual Portuguese is…

A: Is: *"corda bamba"*.

P3:   *"Corda"* means roughly string (rope).

A: *"Bamba"* is the swinging.

P3:   But loose.

P2:   It's to be in a difficult situation, very difficult!

A: Like in the circus!

P3:   But in the circus it's easier, because the thread is distended.

A: It's something I don't know, but my feeling with *"corda bamba"* is something so dreadful! I always remember films, pictures in the circus, where there can be a terrible accident… Gene Kelly!

Bion: It's nearly always the essence of the circus performance is left…

P3:   But like a clown, like a clown!

A: Yes! Exactly! It's not the man who is able to do it, it's the clown, when he wants to do what the acrobats do!

Bion: Why do you disagree?

P2:   I disagree because I don't think it's as hard as this.

Bion: You think?

P2:   I don't think it's as hard as this, it's the idiomatic expression that cannot be very meaningful; in excessively meaning. I can say for instance if you asked me a question, I can say: *"I was in the 'corda bamba' to answer"*.

P3:   It's almost impossible to walk in the *"corda bamba"*, almost impossible.

Bion: I would think that, very often, phrases like that are used so that have become meaningless, or virtually meaningless, but in fact, I don't mean this in this context.

P2:   No, I don't…

Bion: I think they use it, for this express purpose of describing what is really felt to be an extremely dangerous situation.

A: Extremely! It's my feeling.

P2:   I am thinking about the patient's brother, because this patient seems to have come to analysis out of her interest. I know she did, but she came after being part of a group observation. I have had difficulty with some patients that had a prior group observation. They come unable to know anything about themselves.

P2:   I know she did, I said...

A: No!

P2:   Yes, I know she did. She came from an analysis.

A: From another analysis, not a group.

P2:   Yes, I know, but as I said, she gives me the idea, the impression of patients I have had, that have group therapy first and that I had most difficulty to work with; because, they don't know anything, not even, that your servant, your maid knows, they don't! This patient seems to me to be so well defended, she's so dressed with defense that she seems to me always to be most...

[two or three words are incomprehensible]

For instance, when she describes that the boy took her hand and it was so nice, etc... I don't feel that. I think she is acting, performing the good psychologist she is to others. I don't believe very much what she says. Her dying father she doesn't mind. What does she? Dreams? He didn't have anything to eat. Well, it would be very nice, if she would have made food for him. I don't have the idea that this patient uses "Corda bamba" in the real meaning of it; maybe, it has a meaning to her very deeply, but not in the surface. You know, I think she's too much defended to do it.

Bion: I'm reminded very much of an actual dying patient who didn't really believe she's dying, at all!

A: Yes.

Bion: And she spent her time being an awful nuisance to everybody, trying to get them to take her case seriously, but she's the only person who didn't take it seriously.

A: Yes.

Bion: And I would think that this patient's persisting is somewhat similar. Because, I think that she really is afraid of this situation, for which, she is seeking assistance, but, of course, she makes it difficult, because, she can't make up her mind whether to make it clear that it's something that she's frightened of, or whether to make it clear there's nothing to be frightened of.

A: You said something about her father, that is dying and she was not with him. Then, it reminded me that her father sometimes, she used to say, he's very demanding of her.

Bion: Yes.

A: He wants her to go and see him everyday.

Bion: Yes! Now, which father do you suppose this is? Can it be described in any adequate terms? Well, like various human fathers or would you have to consider something like a religious father, a God?

A: Um hmm, yes.

Bion: Who is very exacting and demands daily adoration of...

A: Yes, a God that she hates sometimes, because, he is demanding something
           to eat, the flowers in the vase and so many things... and to be with him.
           But, when it is about the firm, about factory, then he wants the brothers, the
           eldest brother, not her.
Bion: Or demanding that she should be the eldest brother.
A: I think so.
Bion: Which makes it difficult to be the mother.
A: Yes, I think so. Even when she wants some analyst for the family, she has
           to choose the analyst and after she had chosen the analyst, then he says:
           *"Are you sure that he is good? Are you sure that he is the right analyst for
           my daughter or...?"*
Bion: This problem is in which way in this mass of facts that one is to find...
A: Do you think that I could say – following what you said – that she can't
           have pleasure, because she feels guilty! Can I say that, perhaps she thinks
           that her father would not like her because she was not with him, but with
           the other?
Bion: Yes. Well, that's again, a matter of judgment at the moment, because, it
           will keep on popping up, this same story, I think. But the central thing
           seems to me: how difficult it is to be the woman who is able to be the
           good mother, without some sort of moral support. One of the advantages of
           bringing you into this would be: if you dared to be the good mother, then,
           perhaps, she could also dare to be it. But the essential thing is: it can be so
           rewarding to be the good mother...
A: That she thinks that she has not the right!
Bion: I think it's some sort of fear that if she is... she's got to revise her views
           about the mother, all the views about the position of the mother and the
           woman, *vis-à-vis* the brothers and fathers and sons. In fact, review *all* her
           views about the relationship between what we nowadays call the sexes.
P3:   She brought several today, she brought several communications, good
           communications: a good sexual relation, an aspect of the analyst, her smil-
           ing, her smile and that she's different, probably, she's receiving or feeling
           some support from the situation.
A: But, she said something about: *"As an adolescent"*, this sounded to me
           like something – why adolescent only?
Bion: Well, I think that, very often, as an adolescent, the adolescent knows very
           well what it feels like to be a child, because he still is one and he knows
           very well what it feels like to be grown-up, because he is grown-up. But,
           this seems to me to apply to a number of situations which aren't what we
           call adolescence really. But, anyhow, the whole point about the practice of
           analysis is: that you can make up your own mind, from your point of view,
           to what extent the kind of emotional crisis, which you know, comes up to
           the surface, so that, most people notice it. Talk about adolescence and so
           on and so forth... aren't in fact the current events, but, usually, not passing
           notice. It may be that, this situation like it, where there's actually death in

the family pending, it stirs things up, again, in a powerful sort of way, or if she were feeling that she is making the sort of progress, in which she will not be coming for analysis for much longer, then, that can also have a sort of anxiety about it having benefited by the analysis, of really being better off than at the beginning of analysis. It isn't the analyst who benefits from analysis. If you take analysis, if you're fortunate, your patient may improve, but that doesn't help the analyst. The analyst doesn't improve, the analyst is simply so many years older. The parents don't improve if the child gets on well.

A: Don't you think they improve?
          [This was said in a laughing tone of voice]
          I think they improve!
P2:   We think so!
Bion: Well, well, it's quite possible! They do, but it's got nothing to do with their children. Their children on the whole contribute with anxiety, worry and care, financial problems, troubles of innumerable…; but, it may be possible that, as a parent, one somehow or another, succeeds in making something of it. Well, one hopes so!
A: Do you know there is something I want to say about this patient? It is: how she used to dress herself, always with the best things, but, she looks on if it's not the best, but, we know that everything is Italian shoes…
Bion: The best quality. Well, if you have enough money, you can do it!
          [Lots of laughter]

Notes

1 Editor's Note: The Portuguese expression is *cordas bamba*, something like: "walking on a swinging string". That is, in a delicate or difficult position. (see below).
2 That expression is unknown to us.

Supervision D9 commentary

Altamirando M. Andrade

Whenever I read a supervision or discussion led by Bion about a clinical case, I have the impression that many of his theoretical contributions appear throughout the discussion. Not necessarily in a direct manner, but through inferences.

Reading this particular supervision, something interesting came to my mind, which is as if Bion were building hypotheses about the clinical material presented and as if his various questions sought precision in what the presenting analyst felt, perceived, and understood about his patient.

For instance, in the very beginning, Bion asks about crystals, trying to exactly understand the patient's sense of communication. In this way, soon afterwards, the presenter says that the patient would like their relationship to be like a crystal, but it is not yet clear what the meaning of this crystal is. Later, Bion says that it is a rock, but in fact it is a person. It seems that through the questions and the evolution of the session, Bion raised the hypothesis of the patient trying to talk about a personal condition, instead of a rock condition.

The analyst talks about a dream that his patient mentioned during the session. A dream about her dying father who had not been fed. In the dream the patient's sister-in-law tells her that her father did not have his dinner and the patient said she would prepare it. The analyst said the patient did not make a direct association, but started talking about her father and brothers and went on talking about an experience of infant observation about which she had disagreed with a friend. For me, during this conversation, the patient was associating the dream with her dying father and with the baby's mother who was absent during the observation.

The patient seems to alternate between a human and a rock condition. Twice Bion asks where the patient's mother was and if she was absent. It seems that he was using constructions to understand the feelings that the patient was trying to communicate. I will discuss these constructions later.

Bion did not try to grasp the content of the patient's speech, as if he were trying to understand the way the patient was functioning. She has many questions about her dying father, her absent mother, the infant observation, those who are present, but do not care. Moreover, she has some disagreements between herself and the analyst, with her friend about the infant observation and with her husband. What we

DOI: 10.4324/9781003439233-17

do not know is the meaning of these disagreements to the patient, what she wants to convey with the disagreements. Perhaps she has an understanding about the meaning of the disagreements which is different from common sense.

Psychoanalytic work usually consists of understanding the patients' psychic reality and the analyst interprets what he/she thinks is going on. But in this supervision, what we see is Bion trying to build a way to feel the patient, to connect with her feelings. And construction is more appropriate then interpretation to reach such understanding, something described by Freud in *Construction in Analysis* (1937). This was also affirmed by Bion in his book *Two papers: the grid and caesura* (1977) quoted by Junqueira de Mattos (2018) in his book *Impressões de minha análise com Wilfred R. Bion* (Free translation: Impressions of my analysis with Wilfred R. Bion).

Junqueira de Mattos makes some comments about interpretations and constructions and affirms that constructions, due to their polyvalent aspect, are the best way to help patients be in touch with what is going on. The subject was also discussed by Spillius (1988) in her introduction to the book *Melanie Klein Today*. Spillius talks about those Kleinians in favor of constructions and interpretations and those only in favor of interpretations. She says that constructions help patients link their past experiences with those that are current and more useful for being in touch with the patients' emotional experiences. She describes something close to Bion. For those not in favor, constructions move the patient far from the experience of the session's moment.

Bion came from classical psychoanalysis under the great influence of Freud and Klein, but went forward to contact psychic reality, the patients' emotional experiences, both the ones thought about and those not yet thought about. This is a very important leap, because together with the concept of intuition, without memory, desire and understanding in the session, Bion is presenting something that is not sensorial, that is beyond the understandable, but close to the emotional experience which is unknown.

In this supervision, the patient keeps talking about her husband and her wish to buy a house and her husband's opposition to it – he is afraid to spend the money. She goes on talking about the beach she went to with her children and another little boy. There she had an experience with the little boy that she really enjoyed. At this moment, Bion asks about the emotional experience the patient was trying to show to her analyst.

It also seems that the patient has two feelings: one which is of a dying part of herself connected with her dying father and another, which is trying to survive and be capable, such as the analyst who studies and goes to see Bion/Michelangelo. It seems that the patient was close to having feelings of happiness, of being satisfied with her life, irrespective of her dying father and her poor husband, but probably guilt may have prevented the patient from having such feelings.

In his book, *Evidence* (1976), Bion says that it is particularly important that the analyst forges for him(her)self the language he/she is familiar with. He discusses how difficult it is to say something to someone that can touch the feelings of that person, how to be precise about the emotional feelings expressed by the patient, how not to influence or induce moral behaviors or effects.

In this supervision, I perceive almost two superimposed and simultaneous supervisions: one being the clinical material itself and the other being the development of an understanding of the clinical material, the latter appearing in Bion's modus operandi throughout the discussions. How he interacts with the material and with those who are present, the precision he seeks with his questions, his patience to reach an understanding. In fact, we see Bion working as an analyst and supervisor as if he were exposing his ideas by exemplifying them through his own operation: a supervision through the demonstration of the analyst's mind at work.

He takes the discussion of the clinical material as an opportunity to reflect, to think about, but not to teach what to do with the case or with the patient. He is not worried about understanding the content of the material based on a desire/memory perspective, but is connected to feel, to intuit the emotional experience of the patient as closely as possible. I think we can observe this where he says

> Well, what I'm trying to do, again, is to stir something which would get this woman to say, or come a bit nearer to giving some sort of material which would explain why this discussion now.

Bion's theory, as a whole, is not easy to comprehend, and requires continuous reading and studying. Yet, it leaves us with the impression that however sophisticated and elaborate it is, it seeks precisely to reach the human being that everyone has within themselves. In the present supervision, to reach a type of rock that is actually a person.

The interpretations that succeed in making transformations from knowing something to being it (K→O) are those that provoke changes and mental growth. I believe that in the present supervision this phenomenon approaches what Bion means when he states that one notices a search for understanding what and who the patient is indeed, her own truth. To arrive at these interpretations, we notice that Bion gradually builds hypotheses through questions to the analyst and through interactions with other participants. It is almost like a joint construction.

As described by Bianchedi et al. (1973) in her book on Bion's ideas, the analyst addresses the difficult task of capturing the transformations in 'O' in order to interpret them and attempt the K→O transformation in the patient.

At a recent Brazilian Congress in Fortaleza (November 2017), I attended very interesting discussions on the analyst's state of mind in attempting to intuit and interpret the patient's evolutions. Some described the analyst's reverie in the sense of approaching the psychic reality of the patient. Their focus followed the evolutions in the psychoanalytic technique proposed by Bion (1970) in his book *Attention and Interpretation*. And they discuss exactly what, as I understand it, is being discussed in the present supervision. The analytical ability to develop the intuition to approach the patient's psychic reality and thus give an interpretation that ranges from knowing to being.

Bion asks his audience who are present what they assume is the emotional situation that the patient is trying to express to the analyst. I was left with the impression, based on this question and the discussion that followed it, that Bion might be considering a rather primitive state of mind with communication occurring through hallucination. In his conferences and seminars in Los Angeles (April 1967)[1], Bion describes a type of communication through hallucination, *i.e.*, the patient has his hallucination reversed and, through this reversion, 'inserts', through the analyst's eye, a mental state that is impossible to experience with the expectation that the analyst can feel it and understand it. He called this phenomenon 'hallucination as communication'. In the case in question, the patient may be trying to communicate her fear of having to die along with her father. It seems to me that Bion comes close to this subject when he comments that the imminent death in the family shakes things up and that the patient has some anxiety about benefiting from the analysis. This contrasts with the death of her father and her fear of having to go along with him.

I think that part of the discussion that occurred from Bion's question described above was an attempt to understand something, if not equal, at least very close to what the patient experienced emotionally. And that through hallucination, as a method of communication, she informed the analyst of her fear of realizing that her father was dying, but that life would continue, *i.e.*, she would remain alive.

With regard to Bion's long speech that follows A's asking if he thought the patient felt guilty about not attending her dying father, I thought Bion is working through the sessions and their development, and one possibility is that the patient is trying to say or feel that although she is jealous of the analyst because the analyst has a helping hand (Bion) to support her, the patient is wishing for a helping hand that would help her jump from a state of mental block to a state where she can feel and be happy. But for this, she needs to overcome the idea that she cannot be free and happy if her father is dying, her mother is absent, and her husband is poor. Something connected to the idea presented in the infant observation, where her friend was present during the observation, but did not help the baby's mother. So, she is trying to find a way to be happy, but her guilt feelings are not allowing her. This reminds me of the concept of negative therapeutic reaction which, according to Henrique Honigsztejn (personal communication), is when patients feel trapped and unable to evolve, because they think that if they do, they will abandon their parents to their own fate.

In Bion's interpretation, it seems that he takes this subject into account when he proposes something like the understanding that could be offered to the patient: "You seem to be worried about the prospect of benefiting from either your relationship with me or with your family".

Bion raises a point where, for the patient to feel all these feelings, she will need to revise her concepts of mother and father, brother and sister, and mainly the relationship between the sexes. She will have to redesign in her mind those relationships that happened in her life from the beginning. Perhaps this is too much to be dealt with by the patient, because she does not know where these things will lead. They could lead her to experience the disagreements mentioned in the session as between the analyst and the patient and the one between the patient and her husband.

She says that she wants to buy a house, but her husband is afraid of doing so. Afterwards, she says she had pleasurable sexual intercourse with her husband, perhaps meaning that she can have the experience of two different states of mind at the same time. The same happens to the analyst: the disagreements did not prevent an understanding between both of them. But the patient says she is also on a tightrope, swinging as if she were not safe. She continues the session talking about the day on the beach when she had a pleasant time with her children and also the assistance of the boy who helped her jump. She describes this experience as a pleasurable one and conveys the idea that she needs the analyst's assistance to make a leap in her life as I mentioned above. Having feelings evokes a hard and unsafe mental state, but with a creative helping hand, such as God's helping hands through Michelangelo/Bion/the analyst, she can feel safe to take pleasure in her life. This is something that the patient is engaging to reach.

I linked what I just described above with the end of the supervision, where the analyst says that the patient used to dress herself with the best clothes, but functions as if her dresses were not the best. The ragged woman covers the human being that could wear the best of herself.

At the end of the supervision, Bion raises a point that is often discussed among analysts, which is the benefit analysts can have from the analyses conducted. There are some disagreements between what Bion said and what the audience thinks about it. It is always a polemic and interesting point. But I can affirm that a supervision with Bion is an experience that potentially can benefit all involved, including Bion himself!

I would also like to emphasize Bion's important connection with Freud's work. Through his innumerable statements, Bion makes clear the value and understanding he has of the transference work, the role of resistance, the dynamics of the unconscious, and the analytic work as an investigation of unconscious processes. This is obvious, of course, but I think it is necessary to draw attention to the evolution of the psychoanalytic theory and technique proposed by Bion, without departing from the basis that founded Freudian psychoanalytic theory. It may be a fine example of caesura, a concept used by both Bion and Freud.

Note

1 Aguayo and Malin, eds. (2013).

References

Aguayo J., Malin B.D. (2013). *Wilfred Bion Los Angeles Seminars and Supervision*. Karnac Books. London.

Bianchedi E.T., Ginberg L., Sor D. (1973). *Introdução às Idéias de Bion*. Imago Editora, Sao Paulo.

Bion W.R. (1967). *Second Thoughts Selected Papers on Psychoanalysis*. Karnac Books. London.

———— (1970). *Attention and Interpretation*. Tavistock Publications, London.

———— (1975). *Conferências Brasileiras*. Imago Editora. São Paulo, 1973.

———— (1976). *Evidence Chapter of the Book Clinical Seminars and Other Works*. Routledge. London and New York.

Freud S. (1926). *Inibições Sintomas e Ansiedade* – Portuguese Translation by Imago Editora. 1969. Rio de Janeiro.

———— (1937). *Construções em Análise* – Portuguese Translation by Imago Editora. 1975. Rio de Janeiro. (*Constructions in Analysis*. Hogarth Press, 1937).

Honigsztejn H. (1998). *Comunicação Pessoal. (Personal Communication)*. Rio de Janeiro.

Junqueira de Matos J.A. (2018). *Impressões de Minha Análise com Wilfred R. Bion*. Editora Edgar Blucher. São Paulo.

Spillius E.B. (1988). *Melanie Klein Today*. Introduction. Routledge. London.

Chapter 9

Supervision A19

T: He wants to know if he should present a summary of the session or if you could read what's written down?

Bion: Just as you like, whatever you feel is most useful. We have such short time that we must make the best use we can of it. So, pick on the part that you want to deal with.

T: It was a session last Monday, on December, 1977. The patient starts the session asking his analyst if he'd read *"Sagarana"*. It's a book by Guimarães Rosa, a Brazilian writer.

> *It's a very good book and I could perceive, while reading, several very interesting things. It's very good indeed, but I don't read everything because there are parts in it which I'm not interested in, but it's like analysis, isn't it? That helps me understand. The book has many interesting things. There is a part that describes a duel and this part is very interesting indeed.*

Bion: Which describes?

T: A duel, a fight!

Bion: Oh, yes!

T: *"This last weekend I almost didn't go out on Saturday. I was so tired that I had to rest, do you understand? I had to rest".* I (A) said: *"I can't understand what you said very well because you started on one idea and left it and now you're telling me about something else".* He said, the analyst: *"I don't think that communications are clear, they sound interrupted to me as if you didn't finish, I wonder if you noticed that".* The client said:

> *Well, alright… because in Guimarães Rosa's book I read only the part that interested me, I had already perceived that. The fact that I had rested on Saturday made me feel… and that the fact that I rested during the weekend was also important.*

The analyst answered: *"I believe that we are having a fighting duel here, too".* The client replied: *"Yes, but it's very difficult, because what's*

DOI: 10.4324/9781003439233-18

happening is as if we had several situations which are superimposed, one over the other".

Bion: Do you mind being interrupted?

A: No.

Bion: So, if any of us want to get a point clear we can interrupt you and ask?

A: Yes.

Bion: Perhaps each one of us, when you aren't clear about some point, could ask the analyst to clarify, so that we can keep uptodate with what he is telling us. Do you form any opinion about whether you would like to have a patient like this? Would you take him on if he came to see you?

P1:   The patient, how long is he in analysis with him?

T: Almost five years. He's been having a lot, a great deal of difficulty with this client.

He (P1) asks if this difficulty is better now, he (A) says: *"Yes, at the moment yes".*

The dialogs were always like that – and he (A) says it's better now.

P1:   But, I feel I wouldn't take this patient.

Bion: You wouldn't?

P1:   No.

Bion: I asked the question because it's quite a good thing to take advantage of this kind of discussion, because in fact, one always has to make these snap judgments. We have to say to the patient yes or no, when we know very little about it.

T: He (P2) said it's quite early for him to form an opinion if he would accept the client or not, but he has the impression that this would be a very difficult client since he reads Guimarães Rosa and, at the same time, says he enjoys the book, but selects only the parts that interest him; perhaps he would do the same thing with his analysis!

Bion: Yes. I don't think we need mind ourselves to this point about it being too early in the session, because we nearly always have to arrive at these decisions prematurely, but we can ask the question again later in the session and ask the question again at the end of the session. So, you can compare your answers that you give now with the answers you give in ten minutes time, with the answers that you give in fifty minutes time. I often feel about this kind of thing that while one says what you decide, I'm not sure that any of us really decides. I think it's rather like seeing a leaf fluttering down from a tree: it comes down like this and this and this,

        [At this point, Dr. Bion was probably making fluttery movements with his hand]

        and then, lands on the ground one side up: yes or no? So, it would be surprising if one didn't find that one's ideas changed. If you didn't take the patient you'd regret not having taken him; if you do take the patient, you'd regret having taken him. This is the trouble with all these responsible decisions. They always involve choosing what you don't choose. But how nice to be the patient who knows what part of the book to read. He knows what to listen to and what not to listen to. I wonder if he will also be so sure that he'd know at time he's finished analysis. Because if we have difficulty in knowing about this point, it's a difficult thing to believe that the analyst's analysand knows better.

T: He (P2) would like to pose a question to you and it refers to that, for example: after one has a client for five years, if there is not a kind of special dialog between the analyst and the analysand that is quite different from the dialogs they first had, in their first session.

Bion: Yes! it is, I'm sure. Because, we are dealing with a dynamic situation, always changing and patients, all of us, don't like that. We don't like the fact that it's difficult to keep up with our own analysis even. We ourselves are different analysts by the end of a session and so is he, a different person. Superficially, analysis is very slow, it takes a very long time! The closer you are to it, the more it is possible to see how very fast it goes. The problem which is settled yesterday is unsettled today. You can play this game with yourself, for example: here we could write down on a piece of paper the sounds that you hear and then write down at the end of the session again – what sounds do you hear? Like the traffic outside, perhaps a bird and so on... through the list. If you number them one, two, three, four and then, look at it ten minutes later, or half an hour later, or an hour later and write down again the list of what you hear, you'll find the order of the things are different, too.

         Well, we'll refer to this a bit later again, I think.

T: And he (A) said to his client: *"This is a motive, more a motive, another motive, to impel you to try to be clear and say what's happening inside you. On the contrary, if you don't do that, confusion will take place".* After a short silence interval, the client continued: *"When you speak I feel as if it were Zorro's signet mark".* Zorro is that hero that has a horse, a black mask and leaves a mark, Z. Zorro takes a sword and leaves a mark on the things he's been in touch with – *"and I think it happens with you here, too".* He (A) took note of things that occurred to him in his mind, but he didn't tell the client. He's asking if he could say those things to you.

Bion: Yes, sure.

T: He thought about a narcissistic wound, his omnipotence being wounded and not accepting contestation or disagreements, but what he answered to the client was: *"Zorro is a man that brings justice and he fights excesses and injustice".* And the client laughs.

         he, with the sword, he cuts the suspenders of the clothes of the sergeant and leaves the enemy without clothes, that's why I think that you make me feel irritated, because you make me feel without clothes, in the nude. The stories which are in magazines, they always end up like that; perhaps, that's why I am uncomfortable. He asks the analyst: "Don't you agree with me?

Bion: He says that the analyst makes him feel naked?

T: Yes.

Bion: Yes.

T: But he continues and says: *"Don't you remember that the sergeant is a friend of Zorro. Although Zorro makes the sergeant feel, become nude, without clothes".*

Bion: The patient says that?

T: No, the analyst reminds the client that the same person that Zorro attacks is also a friend of his. He laughs a little bit – the client – and says: *"Oh, yes! I quite agree, the sergeant is a silly person".* And the analyst answers: *"Well, a friend for you is a fool. That's why, perhaps, you don't show your feelings of friendship towards me here, in the session".* After that there is a silence.

P3: May I?

A: Yes.

T: He (P3) makes the observation that in the beginning the conversation was more critical, although in different levels, but after the image of Zorro is introduced, it's a more childish image and both the analyst and the client, speak to one another and they are more together in that.

P3: Childish in the sense of infantile symbolism about that patient and the doctor goes on with more ease.

T: Yes, both the client and the doctor enter into an infantile symbolization. Is that what you mean?

P3: Yes.

T: He (P4) would add another question now – continuing his image – if the use of those infantile symbolizations, are containers for the feelings of the patient and his fantasies. If they don't make it easier for the analyst to cope with the analytical situation, like in the beginning of the session, where the feelings and thoughts and words of the patient, were more difficult to reach, because they lacked a container, they were more dispersed.

Bion: What makes it easier or more difficult for the analyst is really irrelevant in analysis! It's too late by then. It's possible to discuss these matters if you go to your own analyst and so on... but, in the practice, in the analysis itself, there's no time for that. You can't even get up and look it up in a dictionary, or look it up in Freud, or an encyclopedia. There's nothing of that kind; you haven't got anything to fall back on. It's only yourself. So, I think that from that point of view, one has to be reconciled to the fact that the time that one can spend on learning is very inadequate and there isn't enough time anyhow. In fact, it's extraordinary to me that psychoanalysts do in fact spend such a great deal of time on conferences, congresses, discussions, trying to learn more! I don't know of any profession – well, possibly parts of the medical profession – that spend so much time on trying to learn their subject.

Now, in the analytic session, one isn't concerned with what one can learn. One is concerned at making such knowledge, as an experience that one's got, at the disposition of the analysand, if he would like to make use of it. One can't say this to the patient, but one knows oneself, that one doesn't know a great deal about this subject, because it's only been going about, after all, two or three hundred years at the most! If you take the whole thing as a... whether it is a... concerning oneself with Sanskrit literature or Plato, Socrates, Kant and so on... Descartes... it's only a little step in this business of learning how to use our brains. How to think, since we are thinking animals!

With regard to the patient, he is even less familiar with it, than we are. So, with this patient, the analyst makes himself at his disposal for a few hours a week to learn something, if he can, from the analyst. So, one tries to tell him, in the simplest language we know, so that he will have a chance of understanding it if he will listen. So, if the patient says, in effect, that he is going to pick and choose what to listen to, one could say:

Well, I hope you will be able to choose the right things. I think that you will turn a deaf ear and a blind eye to what I'm trying to tell you. I can quite see that I might be telling you some things that you don't want to learn, you don't want to hear, you don't want to see. Well, I can't do anything about that, but go ahead by all means.

I have sometimes said to a patient:

Well, if what you are saying is right, then I am the wrong person to come to, you hate being with me here, you hate what I say to you, you don't want to hear it, there's no problem because, as you know, there are plenty of doctors and plenty of analysts and the door isn't locked. So, you can walk out whenever you like. I'm not going to put myself in the position where you can take legal action against me for imprisoning you.

I wouldn't say this to the patient, but I would keep it in mind and I wouldn't want to get myself trapped in that position. I could say: *"Yes, I did try to stop the patient leaving the room through my window"*. Because it's twenty, thirty, forty feet, or whatever it is, from the ground and it wouldn't be safe for him to throw himself out the window; he is free to walk out the door when he likes. But something which is less dramatic, namely: *"Just not listening to what I'm saying is... well, I can't stop it. So, by all means, don't listen if you don't want to"*.

After all, the analyst is trying to show him something which he thinks would be good for him to know. So, I think that whatever the patient says, one doesn't have to lose sight of that fact: we are there to help. So, we don't, in fact, agree with the patient that we are there to cause trouble, or to make things difficult for him. He is free to think what he likes, but we are also free to be what we want to be. I say this because this patient seems to me to want to force you to be the sort of person that would suit him.

Now, the analyst may want to be helpful, but there's a great difference between being helpful, because you want to be and being helpful because you're being forced to be. That makes it much more unpleasant for the analyst. You can always feel this when you have the kind of patient who does that, or the kind of patient who won't allow you to do your work, because you want to do it. Even if you give a correct interpretation you don't get the credit for doing that, because according to him, he's compelled you to give the right interpretation. He simply is denying the fact that this is what the analyst is doing wonderfully.

P1:   Dr. Bion, I wonder if I may ask a question, it's not really joined...

Bion: Sure.

P1:   With this, it's a matter that is coming up... I'm asking again, I'm asking every day. You mentioned a word which I, as analyst, tried to listen. You said the analyst is trying to *help* the patient and we here – I think personally – know too often, that this is not the job of the analyst really. I wonder what you think about it.

Bion: It's because the language is so ambiguous, so many different things are understood by *help*. There's nothing new about this, because the *Oracle at Delphi* was supposed to have carved into the stone: *"Know thyself"*. We're still at it. So, the idea that it is useful or helpful to know thyself is nothing new. In that sense, we're trying to help, because we're trying to say:

> *We will help you to know yourself. If you, my patient, tell me something I will tell it to you back again in a kind of way in which you may be able to see yourself. In that kind of way, I'm trying to be a mirror. It doesn't tell you who I am – that doesn't matter – that's a matter of no importance whatsoever.*
>
> *The only thing that's important here is: you, the patient, can see, by looking at me, who you are! It's the only thing that I can do to help you: to reflect back to you who you are, that you can see in what I say to you an image of yourself. So, if you don't want to know what you look like, I don't mind. You needn't look to me, to reflect you. You can find a different mirror, or if you like, you can look in the pool and see your own image mirrored in the water. That's been done before too by Narcissus, but some people think that it's a deceptive image in the water and it's dangerous to fall in love with what you see.*
>
> *If you fall in love so much that you go into the water, you'll get drowned. If you go into my insides, you might get drowned, but I try not to drown you. I try to reflect you, so that you can see who you are.*

That's another reason why we would like, if we could, not to be a too turbulent mirror, because if we can remain steady, then he can get a clearer
image of who he is; but if we change too much, then it becomes a distorting
image.

You can get this rather exaggerated, if you have an actor or actress who
comes to you for analysis, because they've learnt how to put on make
up. An actor can appear to be an Emperor, a King, a Priest, whatever he
wants. He can put on different costumes and he can see the image in you,
of this particular character. But if you start analyzing such a person, then
you take off their clothes and then they feel naked. This patient has said it:
"You make me feel naked". If he was going to a doctor, he'd say: *"Yes, I'd
like to know the pain"*. *"Oh, no. I'm not going to undress. I don't want to
lie on your examination couch and take my clothes off so you can examine
me"*. Only he is saying: *"I don't want you to take my mental clothes off"*.
In fact, he's asking you to make a deal with him. He will only show you
what he wants to show you, if you'll promise only to see what he wants
you to see. In some ways it's one of the weaknesses of analysis that an
analysand can only get the kind of analysis he deserves.

One doesn't want to appear to make it the analysand's fault, but that's
the plain fact. We can only help people who want to be helped! If the
patient wants me to help him, then I may be able to help him, even if I'm
not a very good analyst. If he doesn't want me to help him, then I couldn't
help him, however wonderful an analyst I was. It's one of the weaknesses
of analysis or anyhow, we can't force a patient to learn. This is forgotten
when a wife urges her husband to get analyzed, or wants the analyst to cure
her husband, or a husband wants an analyst to cure his wife, or child and so
on...

I've said this to a young boy, who said he doesn't want to come and see
me. He's coming because he's got to, because his father or mother has told
him so. I say to him:

> *Well, I can't really help you. I can't see you, because your father or
> mother wants you to see me. But if you'd like to come again, well, I
> shall be here, but this depends on you. Depends on whether you want to
> come, it's your choice.*

This patient seems to me to be making a condition. He'll come to you for
analysis if he can only get the analysis that he wants to get. Well, you can't
very well say to him, but you can bear in mind, that the only cure he'll get
is that kind of cure too.

Well, we have to stop again.

Supervision A19 commentary

Cecil José Rezze

Reading the tape's transcript led me to ask myself what might be the best line of investigation and what Bion might have wanted to communicate through the stimulus of supervision. We will probably have to consider several possible perspectives.

Early in the supervision, the analyst asks how he should present his contribution. Bion answers, *Just as you like, whatever you feel is most useful,* thus leaving the field quite open.

The analyst then describes a recent session in which the client asked him if he had read the book *Sagarana,* by Guimarães Rosa, and states: *It's very good indeed, but I don't read everything because there are parts in it which I'm not interested in, but it's like analysis, isn't it?* And soon after: *There is a part that describes a duel and this part is very interesting indeed.*

The analyst indicates that the direction of the client's speech had changed, and describes his own conclusion: *I believe that we are having a fighting duel here, too.*

This introduction probably made an impact and Bion pointed out: *Do you form any opinion about whether you would like to have a patient like this? Would you take him on if he came to see you?*

Decision – the leaf[1]

Bion discusses the analyst's decision whether or not to take on new a client for analysis. He compares the decision to a leaf that falls from a tree, turning and twisting [he gestures with his hand], and we never know on which side it will fall. This is our situation when deciding whether or not to take on a client. In the last of his *Italian Seminars* (1983, 2014, V), Bion refers to this, and apologizes to the participants for the way he worked – that is, he returns to the allegory of the leaf, saying that during those seminars he had expounded his ideas like a falling leaf and that he himself did not know how it would fall.

It is quite possible that, here in Seminar A19, Bion restricted himself to possible and feasible movements by resorting to a narrative language. Abstractly, we may point out that he formulated what would be Line C in the Grid (dream-thoughts, dreams, myths) (1963, p. 17–21) and that in clinical use we would take into account columns 3 (notation), 4 (attention) and 5 (inquiry). As commentator, my role here is

DOI: 10.4324/9781003439233-19

to find, aided by the Grid, possibly meaningful ideas in the text, i.e., concepts (line F) or scientific theory (line G) (Bion, 1963, p. 22–27).

What was settled yesterday is unsettled today

A participant asks if the situation of the dialogue between analysand and analyst during the session was very different from that of the beginning of the same session. Bion says that indeed it was and observes that his way of working expands in a wide universe. He says: *Superficially, analysis is very slow, it takes a very long time! The closer you are to it, the more it is possible to see how very fast it goes. The problem which is settled yesterday is unsettled today.*

A confirmation of how situations change can be found in the supervision we are examining, but also, perhaps, quite impressively, in the entirety of Bion's works. We might have to examine their 'settlings' and 'unsettlings' that have had a very strong impact on the mental establishment of each one of us and that have led me to ask, "Is the impact of psychoanalytic ideas on our minds negligible?" (Rezze, 2020, p. 19). As an example, we have the transition from "Learning From Experience" (1962) to "Elements of Psychoanalysis" (1963) from which the Grid emerged, so comprehensive and creative that, even today, senior colleagues who study it feel the forcefulness of its novel concepts. However, Bion's last leap occurs when, with imaginative and rational conjectures upon examining adult clients who speak normally, he considers certain manifestations as the mental equivalents of embryonic remains (e.g., the vestigial tail that can be found in adults as a tumor, and the optic and auditory pits of the fetus) and thus deems to investigate the mind in its very beginnings (Bion, 1987, p. 250).

Clinical data and Zorro

(Certain clinical data are repeated here to aid text comprehension.)

The patient begins the session asking his analyst if he had read *Sagarana*, a book by Brazilian writer Guimarães Rosa: *It's very good indeed, but I don't read everything because there are parts in it which I'm not interested in, but it's like analysis, isn't it? That helps me understand. The book has many interesting things. There is a part that describes a duel and this part is very interesting indeed.*

The analyst then observes: *I believe that we are having a fighting duel here, too.*

Later on, after the client says certain things that seem somewhat muddled, the analyst replies, *This is a motive, more a motive, another motive, to impel you to try to be clear and say what's happening inside you. On the contrary, if you don't do that, confusion will take place.*

What follow appears to show that different planes exist between the analyst and the analysand, who asserts, *When you speak, I feel as if it were Zorro's signet mark and I think it happens with you here, too.* And, a little bit later: *With the sword, he cuts the suspenders of the clothes of the sergeant and leaves the enemy without clothes, that's why I think that you make me feel irritated, because you make me feel without clothes, in the nude.*

It seems clear the client is following a path that relates to, but is independent from, the analyst, as confirmed by the expression, *because you make me feel without clothes, in the nude*. Bion stresses this fact and will further develop the episode below.

Not learning

To not learn is a very difficult situation in clinical practice.

In narrative fashion, expressing vast knowledge, Bion points out that we cannot consult a dictionary, Freud or an encyclopedia during analysis, and concludes: *It's only yourself.*

Which brings us to the following quote:

> At no time must either analyst or analysand lose the sense of isolation within the intimate relationship of analysis.
>
> No matter how good or bad the co-operation may turn out to be the analyst should not lose, or deprive his patient of, the sense of isolation that belongs to the knowledge that the circumstances that have led to analysis and the consequences that may in future arise from it are a responsibility that can be shared with nobody.
>
> (Bion, 1963, p. 15)

It is possible that our theoretical knowledge, experience and need to work and offer something to the client may obstruct the vision of freedom, i.e., that the analysand must take the path he or she deems appropriate: *He is free to think what he likes, but we are also free to be what we want to be.*

Although we can, with experience, have a relatively safe view of the paths we can tread, the paths that clients actually follow – and, consequently, the paths that may arise in our mind – are always surprising.

We have come back to the model of the leaf, which throws us back to 'isolation' – *It's only yourself* – and to the painful experience of every analyst, the feeling of loneliness: "Detachment can only be achieved at the cost of painful feelings of loneliness and abandonment experienced..." (Bion, 1963, p. 16).

Significantly, the failure to learn from the experience that unfolds between analyst and analysand is repeatedly stressed by Bion when he insists, *I think that you will turn a deaf ear and a blind eye to what I'm trying to tell you. I can quite see that I might be telling you some things that you don't want to learn, you don't want to hear, you don't want to see. Well, I can't do anything about that, **but go ahead by all means**.*

Bion emphasizes that the client actively participates in not learning, and this leads us to at least two lines of reasoning when approaching his work. If the focus is knowledge, we may relate this fact to the K (knowledge) and –K (minus knowledge) links; if the focus is transformations, we will also have transformations in K and –K and their evolutions.

By pursuing the vertex of the knowledge link (K), the client will develop when a commensal relationship becomes possible in the container/contained relationship, allowing both parties to grow and develop according to the breast and mouth model (1962, p. 90–91). The appearance of –K occurs when the relationship is affected by the envy factor, which prevents a commensal relationship (Bion, 1962, p. 96).

Given the transformation vertex both in the clinical situation presented here and in the description highlighted by Bion above – *I can quite see that I might be telling you some things that you don't want to learn, you don't want to hear, you don't want to see* – we have opted to consider that the analysand acts out the transformation in hallucinosis in an atmosphere of rivalry.

> The general picture the patient presents is that of a person anxious to demonstrate his independence of anything other than his own creations. These creations are the results of his supposed ability to use his senses as organs of evacuation which are able to surround him with a universe that has been generated by himself: the function of the senses and their mental counterpart is to create the patient's perfect world. Evidence of imperfection is *ipso facto* evidence for the intervention of hostile envious forces. Thanks to the patient's capacity for satisfying all his needs from his own creations, he is entirely independent of anyone or anything other than his products from him and therefore is beyond rivalry, envy, greed, meanness, love or hate; but the evidence of his senses belies his pre-determinations; he is *not* satisfied.
>
> (Bion, 1965, p. 137)

I suggest that the characteristics of the description above are similar to those presented under the subheading "Clinical data and Zorro", i.e., they emphasize a duel in which the analysand's actions (C6 in the Grid) withhold from analysis elements that might have denoted his or her nudity. A duel is established with the analyst, who brings it to the fore by saying, *I believe that we are having a fighting duel here, too.*

Two observations by Bion are relevant here. First, "If an object is 'top', it dictates 'action'; it is superior in all respects to all other objects and is self-sufficient and independent of them". Second, "The only relationship between two objects is that of superior to inferior" (Bion, 1965, p. 133).

Regarding transformations in hallucinosis, we should examine the relationship established when we consider the transformations in knowledge that tend towards transformations in O – the ultimate reality (absolute truth, the deity or supreme being, the infinite, the thing-in-itself) (Bion, 1970, p. 26).

Two transformations deserve our attention: T(O) → T(K) and T(K) → T(O).

> [O] can be "become", but it cannot be "known". It is darkness and formlessness but it enters the domain of K when it has evolved to a point where it can be known, through knowledge gained by experience...
>
> (Bion, 1970, p. 26)

It is possible to consider the intersection with O – transformation in O – by means of the configurations of Forms, Incarnation and Phenomena.

Transformations in knowledge – T(K) – tend to transformations in O – T(O) – when a sequence of successive cycles originate from O, which becomes knowable through the product Tβ, which is in turn subject to a second cycle that passes to Tα and then to Tβ – and so on until, in cycle n, TαK passes to TβO (Bion, 1965, p. 163).

In this article, Tpα is a development in hallucinosis that evolves into Tpβ, which is transformation in hallucinosis and, therefore, minus knowledge (–K). This interferes with the chain of transformation in O above.

The development of these ideas is in keeping with Bion's emphasis on clients that do not learn and tend to remain obstructed on the path towards 'becoming oneself', 'O'.

Notwithstanding these considerations, we stress Bion's observation above – *but go ahead by all means* – indicating his willingness and ability to continue to work even under these circumstances.

The mirror

As I wrote this article, I became intrigued with the importance Bion attaches to one's role as mirror – Freud – so as to allow the client see him or herself through the analyst. "The doctor should be *opaque* to his patients and, like a mirror, should show them nothing but what is shown to him" (Freud, 1912, 1975, v. XII, p. 118).

Or, as Bion says, "…memory, desire, understanding [are all] opacities obstructing intuition". Further on, he stresses "… the need for the establishment of freedom from memory, desire, understanding as a permanent, durable and continuous discipline" (Bion, 1992, p. 315).

The corollary of these statements is that psychoanalysis takes place in the emotional experience, in the ever-changing dynamics of the encounter between analyst and analysand.

Continuing… *We will help you to know yourself.*

An important fact, but one that clients often find strange or repulsive, occurs when their goal becomes to enlist the analyst in their private life to solve their or their family's problems, rather than striving to *know oneself.*

Bion implies this when he says patients want the analyst to mold him or herself to their goals: *This patient seems to me to be making a condition. He will only show you what he wants to show you, if you'll promise only to see what he wants you to see.*

When one analyzes such a person, their clothes will come off and they will feel naked. *This patient has said it: "You make me feel naked". If he was going to a doctor, he'd say: "Yes, I'd like to know the pain".* [He would not say,] *"Oh, no. I'm not going to undress. I don't want to lie on your examination couch and take my clothes off so you can examine me". He is saying: "I don't want you to take my mental clothes off".*

Bion adds: *I try to reflect you, so that you can see who you are.*

And he emphatically describes this client's resistance to the possibility *that you can see who you are*, which would lead him into contact with an extremely feared reality – although the core issue is not to 'know' the reality, but to 'be' or 'become' the reality. This transitive verb proposed by Bion (1970, p. 148) implies here the client 'being himself', that is, 'becoming O' – something to which he reacts by saying, *That's why I think that you make me feel irritated, because you make me feel without clothes, in the nude.*

Counterpoints

We would like, if we could, not to be a too turbulent mirror… Soon after, Bion leads us to consider counterpoints in the liaison between the analyst and the analysand.

This passage also leads us to consider that an emotional experience occurs in psychoanalysis between the analyst and the analysand. Bion, by introducing it – *we would like, if we could, not to be a too turbulent mirror* – hurls us into his analogy of the image of a lake reflecting trees – the latter corresponding to O – whereby any atmospheric turbulence on the water may deeply affect the reflected image. In other words, the links of love, hate and knowledge are essential for the transformations of O. Bion hopes to work without turbulence (Rezze, 2022) on the links of love and hate in this relationship of profound liaison with the analysand. This becomes clear when he postulates that, whatever the *analytic situation*, O is available for transformation equally by the analyst and the analysand (author's emphasis) (Bion, 1965, p. 48).

In keeping with the same idea of counterpoint, Bion, in *Elements of Psycho-Analysis*, presents the dimensions of psychoanalytic elements and objects in the realm of the senses, myth and passion. He stresses that "I mean the term to represent emotion experienced with intensity and warmth though without any suggestion of violence […] For senses to be active only one mind is necessary: passion is evidence that two minds are linked…" (Bion, 1963, p. 13).

In the same deep sense of the relationship between analysand and analyst, we find that, "In psycho-analysis any O not common to analyst and analysand alike, and not available therefore for transformation by both, may be ignored as irrelevant to psycho-analysis" (Bion, 1965, p. 48–49).

The atmosphere of joy

With supervisions in small groups, we established a personal relationship with Dr. Bion. This brought joy to everyone. And I was fortunate to have been able to present two clinical situations.

The atmosphere of joy spread to everything involving Bion's visit. One might even ask how much of this joy might be linked to dimensions of a very profound nature, possibly related directly to truth, i.e., to 'authentic pleasure' (Rezze, 2021, p. 307) that brings beauty and wonder to fruition:

> It is easy in this age of the plague – not of poverty and hunger, but of plenty, surfeit and gluttony – to lose our capacity for awe. It is as well to be reminded by

the poet Herman Melville that there are many ways of reading books, but very few of reading them properly – that is, with awe.

(Bion, F, 1981, p. 4)

By using the instrument of 'authentic pleasure', we have sought to investigate a true dimension that goes beyond the common meaning of the word *joy*, hoping to find it in the core of the soul or mind:

> I resort to the poets because they seem to me to say something in a way which is beyond my powers and yet to be in a way which I myself would choose if I had the capacity. The unconscious – for want of a better word – seems to me to show the way "down to descend", its realms have an awe-inspiring quality.
>
> (Bion, F, 1981, p. 4)

Today, over forty years since Bion's sojourn in São Paulo, we clearly see his stay with us yielded many fruits. Many were the works that emerged stimulated by his presence and his own original and creative works. I have the impression that questions remain concerning the disruption of the establishment and its ensuing consequences. Inevitably, institutional officialdom was massively affected by the newly arrived ideas, but I will not attempt to examine this dimension because it is an overly complex issue – not to mention that it might also stir up some very controversial dimensions.

Epilogue

To close these considerations, I would like to highlight once again Bion's observation above – *but go ahead by all means* – typical of his willingness to accept and ability to work.

Note

1   I wish to thank Dr. José Lopes das Neves Neto's reading and valuable suggestions.

References

Bion, F. (1981). "Tribute to Dr. Wilfred R. Bion at the Memorial Meeting", *International Review of Psychoanalysis*, 8:3–5.

Bion, W.R. (1962). *Learning from experience* (London: Heinemann).

Bion, W.R. (1963). *Elements of psycho-analysis* (London: Heinemann).

Bion, W.R. (1965). *Transformations* (London: Heinemann).

Bion, W.R. (1970). *Attention and interpretation* (London: Tavistock Publications).

Bion W. R. (1987). Making the best of a bad job, in *W. R. Bion, Clinical seminars and four papers* (Abingdon: Fleetwood Press). First edition: 1979.

Bion, W.R. (1992). *Cogitations* (London: Karnac).

Bion, W.R. (2014). Italian seminars, in *The complete works of W.R. Bion*, v. IX (London: Karnac). First edition: Borla, 1983.

Freud, S. (1975). Recommendations to physicians practicing psycho-analysis, in *The standard edition of the complete psychological works of Sigmund Freud*, v. XII (London: The Hogarth Press). First edition: 1912.

Rezze, C. (2020). Turbulências. Do aprender com a experiência emocional ao pensamento selvagem, in *Psicanálise: Bion*. Transformações e desdobramentos. Evelise de Souza Marra, Cecil José Rezze, Marta Petricciani (orgs.) (São Paulo: Blucher).

Rezze, C. (2022). From learning from emotional experience to wild thoughts. Turbulence!, in *Bion's Legacy in São Paulo*. Evelise de Souza Marra, Cecil José Rezze (eds.) (New York: Routledge), 33–45.

Rezze, C. (2021). *Psicanálise. De Bion ao prazer autêntico* (São Paulo: Blucher).

Chapter 10

Supervision A15

T: The problem (A) brings is a client who was sent to him with a diagnosis of psychosis. The client was committed to a hospital. At the time, the analyst (A) didn't have time in his schedule to receive the client. Nevertheless, they had an interview, and both agreed to delay beginning treatment until (A) would have time in his schedule. The patient remained at the hospital and he (A) phoned the patient's former analyst, and told him that it was not possible to begin the treatment, because he (A) didn't have any time at the moment, as was already said to the client.

Bion: Who hadn't time?

T: The analyst. So the analyst told the client to wait and he was going to phone him as soon as he had an opening in his schedule, which could fit with the schedule the client could also attend.

Bion: Who had said that the patient was a psychotic?

T: He was referred as psychotic by a psychiatrist and also during the interview (A) had with the client, while the client was still committed to the hospital, where they had their meeting, (A) had the impression that the client had typical psychotic anxiety.

Bion: Yes. I was not thinking about that so much as to simply ask the question: who had said that the patient was psychotic? The psychiatrist? That is one point that I was wondering and the other is: who had he told he was psychotic?

T: Who, the client?

Bion: No, who had the psychiatrist told?

T: Him!

Bion: And what does the patient think that the diagnosis was?

T: He[1] wouldn't know what the client thought he had; what diagnosis or anything. If the client knew he was sick, he doesn't know.

Bion: He must have got to see a psychiatrist, or he must have got to go into a hospital; I don't know whose idea that was.

    [After a very long explanation in Portuguese by the analyst, Dr. Bion intervenes]

DOI: 10.4324/9781003439233-20

I think that the question being answered is a much more difficult one than I'm asking. I'll put it this way: whose idea was it that he was ill or wanted help?

T: He was with another analyst and it seems that that analyst made certain alterations in the schedule, which the (patient) ended up not being able to fit into. So the patient gave up that first analysis. He went home and created lots of problems with his mother and with the analyst that's bringing the case now...

Bion: Why did he go to the first analyst?

T: He (A) doesn't know why he went to the first analyst. But what he understood is that the client wants very much to be with an analyst. (A) doesn't know what happened before, but he could feel while he was with the client, now, that the client wants to be physically present.

Bion: Why I'm asking the question is: where does the idea come from that this patient needs help? Now, we can understand what the analyst and so on did. But the interesting thing is that apparently the patient thinks he needs help. In other words, he's not so mad that he doesn't know that he needs help. There are plenty of people who can be what we call insane, but wouldn't want any help from anybody. They could feel that they were quite all right; but this patient seems, at any rate, to be sufficiently well to know that he's ill.

T: He mentioned a second problem. The client, when he came to the analyst, gave the impression that he idealized and expected a great deal of his analyst. Nevertheless, at the same time, he was sort of mute. He couldn't articulate words to express and get in touch with the analyst.

(A) had already had an experience with a client, a woman, that had a similar mutism and because of that experience, or one may say prejudice, he had the impression that also this client would remain for a long time in silence, mute. The analyst knew his client was an architect, so he suggested to the client that perhaps, if he was having difficulty in using words, or articulate speech, he would like to make some drawings for him.

(A) felt very anxious with this client and that's what motivated him to ask him to make the drawings. The patient accepted enthusiastically and has been drawing in every session ever since. While he is making his drawing, (A) feels the client is in touch with the paper and the drawing. (A) also has a feeling that doesn't occur in his contact with other clients: when he goes to see what the client is drawing, he feels very sleepy. (A) thinks that a kind of ritual has been established, in which the client makes the drawing, (A) then comes close and asks what he's been drawing, the client gives the drawing to (A) and then (A) looks at the drawing and asks what he thinks about what he's drawn. His last words to the client about the drawing change; he may ask: *"How do you interpret this drawing? What have you drawn?"* And in the last session he is speaking about, he asked the client: *"Give a title to the drawing"*.

Would you like to see the drawing?

Bion: Yes, if you would…

[We then hear a noise of paper and the drawing must have been shown].

T: This is the last drawing he made. (A) asked: *"What title would you give to this drawing?"* The client thinks for a while and answers: *"Bestiality advances"*. Then, he asks the client: *"Do you represent the advance of bestiality by a foot that's advancing?"* He replied *"It's not that bestiality is a foot. Bestiality is something that has feet"*. He speaks that quite quickly and then, draws a square around the drawing as if it were a painting. He…

Bion: Whose idea is it that he was an architect?

T: The psychiatrist told him (A) and when they had a contact, the client he referred to it.

Bion: Did the patient agree that he was an architect?

T: He was in architect school.

Bion: Again, who said he was a student of architecture?

T: I had made a mistake saying architect and I corrected for student.

Bion: But, who said he was a student of architecture?

T: From what I understood, it was the psychiatrist that referred the case in the concrete sense at least.

Bion: Where did the psychiatrist get the idea from?

T: He can't remember if the client ever made a reference to being an architect.

Bion: No, it doesn't matter very much, but I'm asking this question, because if it were physical medicine, the patient would say he's got a pain and you could say: *"Yes and where's the pain?"* He could tell you and then you could ask him to take his clothes off, lie on the examination couch and you would try to find out where the pain was. Now, this patient seems to feel that he wants help, so he must have what we would call a pain.

In physical medicine, the doctor would want to know where the source, the origin of the pain was. If the patient said: *"It's my foot that hurts me"* or *"my hand that hurts me"*. You could still say: *"I want to examine you physically in order to see where that pain started"*. You could see that there was a wound in his foot, say, or you could see that there's no wound in the foot, that it seems to be all right. Then you'd have to find the source somewhere else.

Why I'm going on here is: apparently this patient is wise enough to know that he wants help. Now, in a way, I know that the patient doesn't know where the pain started, where the origin of the pain is, nor does the analyst. That's why we have a psychoanalytic interpretation, a psychoanalytic examination. But, one of the points which is so important is to know where did this pain start? Where was the source or origin of it? Including where did the cure start, who thought that the correct treatment for this patient was that he should be a student of architecture.

Now, this point is important from, first of all, a general principal, namely: I think that we, as analysts, will increasingly be asked to come into the story, but goodness knows at what point! Very often when everything else has failed, then they say: *"Send for the psychoanalyst"*. So, we are like helpers, but nobody tells us that they want help until very late in the story! If we were surgeons, we might be called in to operate when a cancer had already passed the point of no recall, when the disease had already got so advanced, that it was past surgical intervention. The same thing applies to psychoanalysts. So, we have to get used to the idea that we are called for too late.

For all we know, we are invited to cure the patient when the patient is already beyond cure. Now, I don't mean that we are in any way unfortunate, because it happens over and over again. People need help but they don't ask for the help until it's too late, or too early. If we were firemen, we could get called up any time by somebody or other who says they thought they smelt something burning and if you get there, you find that there's no sign of a fire anywhere. Or you are asked to save the house that's already in flames and the whole place is almost destroyed. So, we're not really treated any worse than anybody else, but we aren't treated any better either. So, the analyst has to do what he can with the situation which may already be pretty bad.

Now, I could look at this drawing, the one we've just been seeing and say: *"That's a funny piece of architecture!"* This looks like a drawing of a part of the anatomy. If that is the case, then perhaps this patient thinks that the human body is a piece of architecture. He's got a skeleton in much the same way as buildings have skeletons, iron gratings and ferro-concrete skeletons. Put this building in a plan for a building of flesh and blood.

T: This could be the bestiality that the patient refers to? (P2)

Bion: Well, it's very interesting, because the analyst could draw on the assistance of the patient, as he has done, to draw him a picture of it. Now, one has to think again: this patient who's been diagnosed – probably quite correctly, I don't know, I'm not objecting to that at all – as a psychosis is also well enough to know he is ill. That's point number one. He is also well enough to know that the analyst is likely to help him, so he doesn't mind cooperating and drawing the analyst a picture. He doesn't tell him where the pain is, but he draws a picture of it.

T: Isn't it dangerous to consider that a drawing such as this one is really communication by the mind, mental communication?

Bion: I think it is dangerous to consider anything! I think that, in fact, although one doesn't want to follow with these things very much, psychoanalysis is a dangerous occupation. So is being a doctor; so is being a fireman. In all these things, people are likely to lose their lives. Well, we can't be bothered with that, but on the other hand, it is just as well to remember that psychoanalysis is a dangerous occupation. So, it is dangerous whatever you do – if you don't do anything and if you do anything, either way. Now, again, the title of this drawing: what's the title again? What's the diagnosis the patient has given it? What is the diagnosis of that drawing? What did the patient say it was?

T: That the discussed catastrophe, this dangerous event was happening, was walking, between him and the analyst.

Bion: That's not what he said. What did he say it was?

T: *"Bestiality is advancing"*.

Bion: What is that? The name of the drawing? Or the thing of which that is the drawing?

(A):   I think I need help with something like that.

T: He (A) asks if the help that the client is requiring, that the patient is speaking of, if he's talking about the drawing, or talking about himself when he makes the drawing. What kind of help he asks the analyst for and if it's necessary to make a differentiation between one thing and the other?

Bion: That is the problem of the psychoanalyst, the problem of the helper. What are the patient's problems? He knows that he wants help and he seems to think that the person who can give him help is his analyst; but he also knows that his analyst needs help, so he does draw that picture and he says also what the title of that picture is. We could call it the title, or the diagnosis, or the name of the picture. But, again, as far as we're concerned, that picture is of something. Say, if it was a house on fire, one could say that the flames were advancing. If it's a drawing of a piece of human architecture, then it is a state of mind that is advancing: *bestiality!!*

In other words, he does not feel that he's becoming more civilized, more polite, more cooperative, but more bestial. Not more human, but more like the beasts. Well, we're all beasts, we're all animals, although we're rather a peculiar kind of animal and we would all like to become more civilized. So, it's very striking when he says that in his experience it's the beast that is advancing. He doesn't feel that he is becoming more civilized; it means that he's becoming less civilized, more bestial.

Now, we can have another look at this problem to where this started. It's awkward because we're not dealing with the start, we're dealing with where it got to now. So, while we're dealing with the advance of bestiality now, it may have advanced too far already. It would also be useful to know where it started, where the origin was, because, perhaps if we knew that we could stop the origin from feeding the advance!

If we were again dealing with a fire, it would be important to try to contain that fire, to prevent it spreading more, but also, it is important to know what was starting it, or what was feeding it. If it was, say, physical ailment which was advancing, it would be useful to know where the source of the infection was. So, if it is bestiality that is advancing, it would be useful to know the origin of this bestiality. So, the problem that we are up against is both: to stop its spreading further, but while doing that, also guessing where it started. So that, while one can try to help the patient, one could also try to find where the person who was not trying to help the patient was; who or what is helping the advance of bestiality.

Now, in fact, I think that the analyst asking the patient to draw this picture is helping to contain the spread, because drawing is quite a civilized procedure. It's got a long history! Artists and painters have also got a long history. They even go back to cave drawings, which we all know. So, in the patient, one has got the signs of something that is a long history, is right up-to-date and we come into the story very late. So, I think it is quite helpful to mobilize his capacity to paint or draw. That does give him a bit of exercise on being civilized. There's still this question of where it originates, where the bestiality originates. If you look at the cave paintings at Lascaux, for example, there you can see the artist's drawing of where the bestiality got to, so far.

I'm afraid we've got to stop for today.

Note

1 Editor's Note: Presumably, the 'Him' and 'He' in these next two comments by the translator refer to the analyst, (A).However, the transcript is somewhat ambiguous and we are left to assume that the ambiguity extended to the listening audience. We have left that ambiguity in this printed version of the transcript, on the assumption that it was a part of the emotional experience of the supervisory moment and therefore potentially a reflection of something in the treatment relationship that was being conveyed to both Bion and the audience.

Supervision A15 commentary

Deocleciano Bendocchi Alves

This supervision took place in the past. In my commentaries, I am bringing it forward to present time. What Dr. Bion thought and said is said and done and cannot be changed. My commentaries will be made based on Dr. Bion's final contributions and the clinical material stimulated in me, expounding my current ideas in the belief that they may incite new ideas in you, the reader.

1 – In considering the first part of the material, I surprisingly caught myself questioning why analysts would put forward for supervision a patient with so many difficulties and in relation to whom the analysts had so many questions as to how to conduct the analysis. The supervision ought to be a time when two psychoanalysts could discuss human situations lived in the day-to-day experience of those who seek their help. If we are not idealised as sages, cloaked with authority, we could have a sensible and creative discussion.

2 – The questions posed by Dr. Bion have a vital importance to all of psychoanalytical work. They remind us to always question all information that comes to us, as well as all apprehensions we glean from our observation. The latter must be refined and free of any prior knowledge, independent of its source. Intuitive knowledge coming from careful observation carries more weight than already packaged knowledge. The latter is constrictive, offering only an illusion of solid ground based on 'hearsay evidence' or diagnoses made from a psychiatric vertex.

3 – I believe that any analysand who comes to us for guidance conceives an idea of the work we do and the professionals we are, as well as an idea of who and what he or she is. This conjecture may be formed or not, prior to or in the course of the analysis. It is thus up to the analyst to abstain from assuming *a priori* any such conjecture in the mind of the patient with respect to either his work or himself. The analyst's desire to have the patient speak, cooperate or come into contact with the analyst is a phenomenon tantamount to expecting an ideal patient.

In regard to the patient who doesn't speak, mutism is in its essence a matter for observation and it must be observed. When we learn in the supervision that the psychoanalyst was prejudiced against mutism, we perceive that the analyst's observational perspective was distorted. This prejudice deprived the analyst of

DOI: 10.4324/9781003439233-21

two essential conditions necessary for observation and psychoanalytical intuition: first, the suspension of disbelief and second, the maintenance of an openness to the unknown. The latter I call an undistracted stance – after the term coined by the biologist H. Dingle – which I feel is an essential psychoanalytical quality.

If we pay careful attention to the material, we find that the certainty afforded by prejudice interferes with creativity and dampens the psychoanalyst's and analysand's 'urge to exist'. This dampening tends to skew the analytic discourse towards that which is conscious and blurs one's ability to grasp the fragmentation of the emotional experience, thereby stifling it.

4 – It was mentioned that the analysand gave his own mother a lot of trouble. I believe this to be a critical point to be examined. What kind of problems were these? Who pointed out these problems? As we do not have much to go by in the material, let us suppose it was emotional turbulence and that this turbulence was not contained by the patient, who acted out his anguish. I suggest that the trouble he caused his mother reflected the eruptions of unbearable fantasy and anguish that invaded his mind, his articulate speech, causing his behaviour to become conventionally unacceptable.

It is in order to accommodate the conventionally unacceptable, that leads patients to be isolated in a hospital. This response is considered acceptable to the social group as it attempts to annihilate the patient's disruptive impulse. On the other hand, there is a socially acceptable convention that the patient needs to be cured and in order to be so, psychoanalysis is then deemed to be the acceptable means. But these statements refer to the social group and not the patient himself. The question is: Did the patient wish to undergo psychoanalysis or did he even want help?

Could we suppose that his actions were part of the asking-for-help process, prompted by an uncontrollable transformation that was going on inside him. What kind of transformation was this? Although his way of asking for help was unusual, did it show that the patient recognised that he needed help? Did he authorise someone to help him? Was this someone the psychoanalyst?

I believe that at this point what is required of a psychoanalyst is to be passionate about analytical psychology and capable of observing and allowing for the development of the session. If a person needs help, he expects to find someone who is able to help. He needs an analyst who is passionate about psychoanalysis and not just any professional in the field. Thus, the analyst's intentions become a necessary part of the clinical material.

During their lifetime, every individual needs to be seen. How can he be seen? He needs to be seen, heard, felt, touched and smelt. The psychoanalyst must also be seen. Therefore, they both need to become sensorially seen and because they are seen, heard, touched, smelt and felt, they exist in the world. But how can one distinguish the individual differences? If there is an impulse to be seen, how does one satisfy the intrinsic need to be? How does one satisfy the 'urge to exist'? How can one be seen more completely? In other words, in our existence how can we make what we feel and think apparent? In regard to what we call psychic experience – and proclaim it as such – THE ACTUAL EXPERIENCE NEVER APPEARS, BUT RATHER, WHAT WE COME TO OBSERVE IS WHAT WE THINK OF IT AND EXPRESS IN THOUGHT. If in animals emotions are expressed through the characteristic sound of each species, human beings during their evolution were also able to develop a verbal capacity to express what they feel and put thought into words, giving it meaning. Human beings can also reflect upon their psychic experiences.

If the patient 'created problems' for his mother, it seems to me that he was unable to find another way to say what he felt or thought. We could perhaps conjecture that he was in a primordial state of mind. How could he externalise his emotions and feelings? Animals make noises: they growl, bark, meow, low, etc. These are primitive forms of expression. During the evolution of the order of primates that gave origin to humans, there must have been a stage when noise predominated as well as actions in order to express emotions and primitive affectionate needs. But then our species evolved to the next level and learnt to express themselves through speech, which was when the incipient ability to think emerged. As a result, human beings began to effectively appear with perceptible sensorial aspects and the capacity to manifest thoughts concerning their feelings and emotions, as well as to base their thinking thereon, which preceded and directed their actions.

During my professional life I have observed that when this devastating primordial anguish emerges, a situation of persecutory delusion sets in, resulting from the senselessness that follows from the patient's failure to give voice and meaning to his suffering. Very often, this senselessness extends to any treatment including psychoanalysis, which then become a threat and the patient, feeling persecuted, merely defends himself.

Going back to the session, there is one fact that in my viewpoint is relevant. On examining the drawings, the analyst asks questions instead of allowing his observation and intuition to evolve to a point where he could express them in the space that was created, based on the drawings. The analyst remarks that the patient is in contact with the paper and the drawing. Differently from the analyst, I believe that the patient is in contact with his inner world of feelings and anguish, and needs a spokesperson to express them in an elaborate form; to transform them into thought. The ritual seen by the analyst under supervision is, I believe, a religious ritual in which rationalisation is taking the place of intuition.

5 – The only verbal expression present in the session under discussion is, "THE BESTIALITY ADVANCES". Soon after, correcting the analyst, he says, "IT IS NOT THAT BESTIALITY IS A FOOT; IT IS SOMETHING THAT HAS FEET". To which bestiality does this refer? Whose is the bestiality? The analysand's? The analyst's? Or both? Is bestiality a quality of the psychiatric internment or something that is evolving? Does the bestiality refer to the emotional turbulence he is experiencing? Are these the primordial feelings and anguish he feels advancing inside him? Does the patient feel that the bestiality in this

session is increasing due to the analysand's and the analyst's lack of insight or receptivity? Does he feel that his anguish is being returned without elaboration?

We very often say, "placing a foothold on something". What foothold is the patient gaining? If he has a foothold, I believe that something is still maintaining his grip on reality before he loses the capacity to think about his psychic experiences. The foot squelches the 'beast's' footprint but also fastens it to something: the awareness of the need for help, even if he is in danger of not being able to get it. When the patient draws the square, which to me seems like a selected fact surrounding the foot, he is depicting pictorially the need to contain the beast that is advancing. The baby needs the breast to contain its cannibalistic anguish. Our patient needs a framework to contain an advancing cannibalistic beast. I believe that his pain derives from the absence of an internal system that gives him the necessary confidence to challenge this bestiality. The bestial feature is manifested in the impossibility of establishing verbal communication of any kind, at any level.

Bion makes reference to the Lascaux cave paintings. Experts conjecture that at the time Lascaux was decorated, Europe boasted some fifty to one hundred thousand inhabitants. Who painted the cave? Was it a single artist or several? We still have no answers to these questions, but what we do know is that it was more than 20,000 years before the Shakespeare period when a man who could express and ponder human emotions and feelings in the form of poetry with majestic expressivity came into existence. In the Lascaux period, there is no artistic manifestation represented by words. If we check out the Lascaux and other caves in the Dordogne area, there is not a single representation of human beings in such elaborate form as the animals; all the human figures are rudimentary. What did these animals in movement signify? Were they an expression of fear, reverence or higher forces? We do not know, but if we examine the Egyptian drawings and compare them with those at Lascaux, the latter have movement and a slight perspective whereas the Egyptian drawings are static and lack perspective. The Egyptians were far more civilised, but why was their art so formal? They could write and were socially organised and yet their art was stiff and formal. Could this lead us to conjecture that religion thwarted its spontaneity?

Is the patient afraid of the increasing bestiality, the advancing bestiality? Does he feel threatened by his inability to put his emotions into thought? Is he not capable of thinking and articulating thought into words? Or is he moving towards a bestial expression of his inner life?

In my viewpoint, bestiality was a factor present in the session given that there was no transformation of the sensorial into verbalisation that would assuage his anguish and provide some insight into his psychic life.

In conclusion, I would say that something was evolving during the session. It did not evolve into an insight, but rather to a manifestation of a nameless terror, derived perhaps from the analysand's impossibility of being helped in gaining greater knowledge of the nature of his pain. Here we have a patient who is suffering because he feels he is losing his awareness of being an individual and returning to the darkness of psychic indifference, i.e. to his disappearance: the return to bestiality.

Referências Bibliograficas

Arendt H., Vida do Espírito (1995), *Tradução de autores varios*, pag. 26, Ed. Relume-Cumará, Civilização Brasileira, Rio de Janeiro.

Bion W.R., *Cogitations* (1994), Dream-work-alpha, pag. 63–68, Karnak Books, London, 1994.

Bion W.R., *Cogitations* (1994), May 1970, pag. 314–315, Karnak Books, London, 1994.

Deleuze G., *Bergsonismo* (1912), Tradução de Luiz B.L. Orlandi, São Paulo, 2012, Editora 34 Ltda, Sao Paulo.

Dingle H. (2010). Great migrations. *National Geographic Magazine*, 28–50, November.

Freud S., *Escritorescriativos e devaneio* (1908–1907), pag. 149–158, Standard edition, versão Brasileira, Rio de Janeiro, Imago Ed.

Chapter 11

Supervision A35

A: I hope that my English will be understood by everybody. I would like to bring material about a girl who is eighteen years old. She's been in treatment with me since last November. I saw her parents previously. They told me that they are very worried about their girl, because she refuses to eat. She had been in treatment – in psychoanalytic treatment before – for almost one year; she stopped. She had a man as a psychoanalyst.

Bion: Did you know the psychoanalyst?

A: Yes! Very well.

Well, when she stopped her treatment in October, she asked her father to look for a new doctor again – but she said to him that she wanted a woman, not a man.

Her illness, apparently, began when she was fifteen years old. Apparently, she only wanted to not be so fat – but she wasn't fat, really. She is a beautiful girl, and she had always had a beautiful body – as her parents told me, and as she told me herself. But she said that for esthetic reasons she would like to be thinner.

On that occasion, she had a boyfriend that lived in another town far from here; well… she finished with him and only writes to him.

Bion: She finished with the boy?

A: With the boy. Since then, her diet had become stronger; suddenly, she almost stopped eating… When she eats, she prepares her food herself. For example: she can eat only one egg, a little fish – prepared by herself. It's unbearable: her impression is that her stomach is full. She cannot stand this feeling. Then, she also began to take laxatives – strong laxatives; some days she would take fifteen capsules. For her, as she told me, that drug… well, she feels that she's addicted to the pills – the pills for her are as a tranquillizer. When she takes the laxative, she feels more secure.

Well, when I saw this girl, my feeling was of… I felt sympathy for her. She shook my hand formally and said to me in a tense voice – transmitting her emotion – that she wanted to be treated, because she is afraid that she could not stop something – that she doesn't know what it is – but that it can kill her.

DOI: 10.4324/9781003439233-22

Bion: Well, can we just stop for a moment? You don't mind me interrupting you and asking questions?

A: No, certainly not!

Bion: Now, as this patient came to see you, and you heard that story from the patient, what impression would you get? What would you think is the central point about this? The main thing? Was there any part of that story, which you would underline, as giving a clue to the whole story?

P: That she has to cook her own meals. I am saying that may be the main point you asked about. She only ate the food she prepared by herself.

Bion: Does anybody else feel that there's any point that they would want to follow up more?

P1:   She comes there for having something inside her.

Bion: What do you think it is?

P1:   So many things…

Bion: I'm not saying that you've got to say to her necessarily, but simply from the point of view of yourself, what would be your impression?

P1:   One thing, she can't bear to have the analyst…

A: May I proceed?

Bion: Yes.

T: He (P3) has the impression that the patient has the necessity to feel herself constantly empty inside; empty.

A: Well, now it reminds me… after our first contact, when we began our analytic sessions, she told me that… well, she shows to me how full she is of aggressiveness, and how people sometimes feel that she's so arrogant… She cannot convey to other persons or people, an impression other than coldness. So, my association was, in that moment, that she cannot… she must be empty. But, what she showed me was that she felt that she was full of hate and aggressiveness, I don't know…

Bion: One point about that is that to take up this particular point: that she feels very beautiful, in the sense of a star is very beautiful. It's a long way away… it glistens like steel… like a light… like diamonds… but those are very beautiful, very far away… and useless. Like a beautiful star in the sky. But, the same thing also applies to the woman who is so beautiful, that nobody would dare to approach her majesty, this beautiful queen. If you did approach her, you'd find that she was sterile… like the beautiful star that is useless. This is the beautiful woman, whose majesty doesn't allow you to get near to her. But, if you could get near to her, then you would find that she was sterile. In some ways, she knows that. That's one part of it. The other side of it is this: this fear that she could become pregnant; then her beautiful body would just swell up; she'd no longer be athletic, like a boy, like a beautiful boy or girl. She'll no longer be in a position to compete, in a sort of Olympic game. So, there's fear of becoming pregnant, and there's the fear of being sterile, cold, unapproachable – both of them together.

A: Of what?

Bion: Both together. There's still this point. Of what is this thing that she is afraid of? That's what I would draw attention to. The thing that she has mentioned, I think accidentally, because she isn't aware of it, but what in fact terrifies her is *this force, this urge*.

T: She (P5) wants to give an opinion, she thinks the patient is afraid of being poisoned and that's why she prepares her own food.

Bion: Certainly, that's only a part of the story. The story, which I think really centers on the feeling that she is a person of no importance, and she is the slave of *forces* that don't care what happens to her, anyway.

A: Well, may I proceed?

Bion: Yes.

A: Well, when you told us about pregnancy… I had during a session this idea; I told her about pregnancy when she told me that she cannot feel her stomach full, she then brought me a dream: that her female dog was pregnant – I don't know if the term is correct, excuse me – that the dog was delivering little dogs. The patient told me that, during the dream, she felt that her dog was feeling the same feeling that she feels when she evacuates some…

Bion: It's entirely true.

A: But, then she said: *"Well, in the dream, when I* (the patient) *went to take the dog, I saw that the dog was transformed into sandwiches, in food".*

So, I think that this material was important.

Bion: It's denying a feeling that there is an urge to exist. Now, it is difficult to describe, because this urge to exist is felt to be something that doesn't care whether you are an animal, or a human animal, a dog, or a bitch, or a beautiful woman. In fact, it's entirely indifferent, and from this point of view, there's a feeling that the urge to exist, makes use of creatures like dogs, human beings, to perpetuate its existence; but doesn't mind what happens to the thing or person that it uses in the process. So, it's a matter of complete indifference; it's a force that's completely indifferent to what happens to the mother. The mother might die; the offspring might be eaten up, but all in the service of this power, this force of existence, this power to exist. So, she can be afraid of being used, simply as a means to perpetuate existence, as if one could say:

> *I don't mind what it is, more plants, more dogs and more humans. I don't mind a bit what it is. I don't care what happens to the plant, or the bitch or the mother… so long as I can perpetuate my own self, my own urge to exist.*

So, the patient fundamentally, is terrified of being a slave to that *urge to exist*.

I could perhaps make it a bit clearer, by consenting to the opposite of that. In some sense, the opposite of it is the analytic view, which is based on a respect for the individual. In this respect, our own attitude is based on this kind of philosophical belief: in the importance of the individual. It's based on the kind of respect for the individual person. The *force*, to which I'm trying to draw attention, doesn't mind what happens to the individual. One can put it like this: if the human race blows itself out of existence, with a neutron bomb, the force to exist wouldn't mind in the least. I would just be one more discarded experiment. So, it is a matter of indifference, as to what happens to the human race – or any other race, provided the urge to exist goes on... in some form or other.

P2:   You mean anything but yourself?

Bion: This idea of yourself, myself and so on... is based on respect for the individual. Politically, it means that we think the state is for the benefit of the individual, not the individual is for the benefit of the state. But, this force has no respect for the individual at all. This force doesn't mind, whether you are a human being, a dog, or a bacillus, or an algae, for that matter, as long as existence goes on... what happens to the individual existence is a matter of indifference. Now, I don't think it's the slightest good saying that to the patient. I think that's something that is simply useful – it would be useful to me, if I was analyzing this patient – but, I would expect everything to fit into that basic theory; I'll expect it, all the time, to crop up, where this patient is waging war against this force wanting to remain a person, wanting to remain a beautiful person, and so forth... and doesn't like being a slave to that power.

A: To?

Bion: To that force, that power, that energy.

A: Well, now other ideas came to me... She always complains that she feels that her mother is completely indifferent to her. She was three months old, when the mother became pregnant again, and suddenly stopped her breast feeding. This girl, till today, complains against this event; she accuses her mother – that her mother was badly depressed on that occasion.

Bion: Was what?

A: Depressed, on that occasion, when she was three months old.

Bion: It's convenient also to be able to blame the mother, but, in fact, I think that the fear is that the mother herself is a slave to the existence, to this urge to exist, so that she can produce a baby – but it doesn't matter, she can produce another one, straight away. Whether it's good for her or bad for her makes no difference; she has to go on producing babies, in the same way that a bitch has to produce puppies, and a bitch has to produce puppies, in the same way that a sausage machine produces sausages: they'll just get eaten up. In short, one could say: it's a blind force, which has no concern for what happens to the individual at all; infant mortality, maternal mortality, none of those things matter – none, in the least.

A: About her father, she tells me she feels that she must be a beautiful daughter, a tender child, always smiling. She also feels that her father invades her privacy – that her father controls her, demanding things. But, at the same time, she tells me that maybe it isn't true what she tells me, because maybe it is only her feelings; maybe her father is suffering with her illness; he's only preoccupied with her situation. But, what she feels is that he invades her. When he stands up and puts his hand upon her, she rejects him and cannot tolerate any manifestation of tenderness.

Bion: Again, I think that the same feeling exists in regard to her father and mother. The father also is really felt simply to be an instrument in the progress of existence. I repeat this word existence, but I'm really trying to describe something that has got no human characteristics at all. So, from that point of view, it can be that the father, again, is a slave to the same power, and these little rules about incest and so forth, don't count. So, it, this force… if the father submits to that force, then he will, unhesitatingly, seduce his daughter and want to seduce her into producing more babies. It's almost like: more causes, more babies, more bees, more plants, and more people; but, quite regardless of what happens to the people or the individual plants.

If one looks to it historically: there was a time when pharaohs, for example, had incestuous relationships as a privilege. Nowadays, it isn't fashionable for parents to have incestuous relationships with their offspring, but I think that all that is felt to make very little difference; incest still exists, and the force behind that is really felt to be very powerful; it's much more powerful than what we might be able to call sex or sexual pleasure. It shows us, simply, minor things that we are aware of, as human beings. The fundamental thing is: that this force is completely indifferent to the individual, plant or animal. So, I think that the patient would be, first of all, afraid that the analyst would be just one more of these objects, which is a slave to this power – or alternatively, the analyst is also engaged in a hopeless war for individual existence against this massive force. In fact, I don't think that she has found a way of mobilizing anything against that kind of omnipotent drive.

A: Can you repeat this?

Bion: She can't mobilize any resistance against that omnipotent power.

A: Yes, and…

P2:   Do you think that this is her problem, or not?

Bion: I think that all of her problems are related to this one. All the individual problems are really aspects of the same thing. It's like looking at one's hands, if you look at them through a microscope, you see individual cells – but they're not very important; they only add up to a total totality that you call a hand or a body. So, the individual piece of life – whether it's a dog, or a plant, or a human being – is simply one little particle in this total existence. The force doesn't mind what happens to it anymore than you mind what happens to one of your cells, your skin which is shed; you don't even know that you've worn it out.

A: She has a… Well… I interrupted at least…

P2:   Well, that force, when I said if her problem was that she feels not capable, not able to resist this force, or not... I think I understand what you said about this force. But in her case, in that girl, her problem isn't the existence of this force, is that? Because this is something that she knows... or she doesn't know...

Bion: She doesn't know it in any conceptual form. She doesn't know what this force is. For example: she probably thinks she is beautiful, because she wants to be beautiful – she goes to beauty parlors; I have no doubts in all that. In fact, again, I think that the beauty of the individual has got very little to do with her, and is simply a way that would lead her to be seductive. Somebody would... something would want to have intercourse with her, and she herself, unaware, is aiding the process. The more beautiful she is, the more likely she is to be used as a mate. So, her problem in a sense is how to be beautiful, but unapproachable, on the grounds that she is so beautiful, so majestic, that nobody would come near her. Indeed, you can find examples of it yourself.

          One is sure to come across the man or the woman, who is so beautiful that they are unapproachable. They are people who can act on the stage, like kings and queens, and nobody can approach. It's a sort of defense; it's not a very good defense, because it also attracts people. You can almost certainly find situations where men have married some extremely beautiful woman and have been living miserably ever after; because the beautiful woman, so lovely, so unapproachable, is actually sterile, she's cold, it's impossible to have any warm dealings with her. It would be very surprising if you don't come across a man, who complains of just that situation, that they married a beautiful woman, or married a beautiful man, and he's impotent. You expect to be fulfilled and you aren't – whether you are the man or the woman. You could be either side of the occasion. But, of course, mind you, there is a difficulty: you can't, very well, choose an ugly man or an ugly woman as your mate. That would not solve the problem.

A: She, if I understood, speaks very much about a force – about an unknown force inside her. Some days, she tells me: *"I know that I will only recover my health, when I decide that I want to be well again"*. She puts things in such a manner that I think: *"How can she be so certain about what she is saying?"* As if she could control her illness, decide or not about her illness...

Bion: She may not be able to do that, but she can control you! She can get you to agree with her that she has power, but she hasn't. She would like to have the kind of analysis in which the analyst would say: *"Yes, you're quite right; you have got all that power, you are potent, you are omnipotent even like a very powerful king or queen"*. In fact, she couldn't, because she knows she isn't. She's the slave to forces that she can't control. It's true that she can locate some of them from inside herself, but she herself, would be liable to become pregnant in response to a kind of urge from inside, to find a mate. To find something, that would impregnate her. Though it isn't only inside her, it's outside her as well. Plenty of people who would say: *"I can't think why you don't marry… a beautiful girl like you, you haven't got a husband, why not?"* and so on… She's almost sure to have plenty of people who have been saying that kind of thing to her. I'm sure that you can meet people who will resist: *"You know, you're very gifted. It's such a pity you aren't doing this or the other thing, when you are so fitted for it, so gifted".* But they don't, they resist. People who are extremely gifted will refuse good jobs, because they are afraid that the very gift themselves will be exploited in a way which is indifferent to them.

A: She has a physical problem – endocrinological problem – she's very thin, but she doesn't want to tell me what her weight is. She said she doesn't want anybody to know. When she goes to the doctor, she's very anxious; she tells me that she doesn't tolerate the fact that he can do something for her.

Bion: Doctors very often say: *"Right, that is your trouble. Now, will you take off your clothes, and get on the examination couch".* That's what they are afraid of. But, analysts are doing the same thing, analysts say:

> *All right, now I want to examine you; I shall want to see you four times, five times a week and we'll carry on this peculiar kind of discussion, which I call analysis; which, in fact, is an examination of the mentality or character or personality of a person.*

One of the problems of a patient like this is that the patient feels they haven't got a character, they haven't got an opinion, they've got no minds or opinions of their own – that they're frigid, that they have got no feelings of their own. So, they're frightened of that examination, whether the examination is only a temporary affair, like seeing a doctor, or a longer one, like an analysis, or still a longer one, which occurs if you go as far as to marry somebody. Because when you are marrying or when you are married to a wife or a husband, you're sure to find out an awful lot about each other. There's no experience that's quite like the marriage experience, for laying bare the personality in all it's nakedness. I am afraid that we have to stop…

P: What about the chances of her having a psychotic, a clinical psychotic breakdown?

Bion: Not yet, but later, when she's made more progress, something of which the patient is frightened now, and will be very frightened when it happens – and they'll also want the analyst to be frightened. But, what is more, they'll mobilize a lot of people to say: *"What have you been doing to that beautiful, gifted girl? She was wonderful, she was all right, till she came to see an analyst".*

See, you'll have all that coming…

P: Probably she'll come up with another analyst…

Bion: Exactly, but she'll have to go out and find another one first.

        [General laughter]

        I think we had a very interesting case, but you will sure have plenty of trouble.

A: Yes.

Supervision A35 commentary

Juarez Guedes Cruz

Clinical material

Bion supposedly said once that psychoanalysis was a way to offer clinical answers to problems that philosophy had always presented to the human being (Chuster, 2018). Put another way: for centuries, philosophy sowed a culture with thoughts and questions that found, in psychoanalysis, thinkers to think these thoughts from an intrapsychic point of view. I think the material presented in this supervision—and Bion's approach—are eloquent demonstrations of that. At the beginning of the presentation, Bion is attentive to the comment that the patient wants to be treated because she is afraid of not being able to stop something, unknown within her, that could kill her (p. 1). *"That's what I would call attention to"*, Bion says, *"… what actually terrorizes her is this force, this desire. The feeling that she is a person of no importance and that she is the slave of forces which don't care what happens to her"* (p. 3).

Soon after, Bion relates this something, unknown, and feared by the patient, to an *'urge'* – imperious force, intense desire – which, in his words, is an irresistible stimulus

> *… which doesn't care whether you are an animal or a human animal, a dog, a female dog, or a beautiful woman.* [A persuasive and embarrassing force that] *uses creatures like dogs, human beings, to perpetuate its existence but doesn't care what happens with the thing or person used in the process.*

He adds:

> *It is a force completely indifferent to what happens to the mother. The mother may die, the offspring may be eaten up, but all in the service of this* existential *force. (…) She* [the patient] *is afraid of being used simply as a means of perpetuating existence…*

> (p. 3/4)

In the above quotation, I underlined the word 'existential' because it is linked to my approach in this commentary and in Sartre's book, *Nausea*: the relationship

DOI: 10.4324/9781003439233-23

between Bion's understanding of this girl's pain and the conflicting existentialism announced by Sartre in his romance "*Nausea*". But let us not hurry; let us see how Bion continues:

> ... *the patient is terrorized of becoming a slave to this urge to exist. (...) The force, for which I'm trying to draw attention to, doesn't care about what happens to the individual. We can put this way: if the human race blew itself out of existence with the neutron bomb, the force to exist wouldn't mind in the least. It would be just one more discarded experiment. Therefore, it is a matter of indifference to what happens to the human race – or any other race, as long as the urge to exist continues.*

(p. 4)

Further on, he comments:

> ... *this force has no respect for the individual. This force does not care whether you are a human being, a dog, a bacillus, or an alga, as long as existence continues... what happens to individual existence is a matter of indifference.*

(p. 4)

Bion adds that he would not say any of this to the patient, but finds it very important that the analysis reaches the point in which the adolescent "... *is engaged in a war against this force; wishing to continue being a person...* [who] *does not like to be a slave*" (p. 4). Slave to a compulsion that, in the patient's fantasy, her mother is also submitted to:

> ... *fear that the mother herself is a slave of the existence, of this urge to exist, so that she can produce a baby – but this is not important, she can produce another one soon after that. Whether this is good for her or bad for her does not make the slightest difference; she must continue producing babies, just as a dog must produce puppies, and a dog must produce puppies the same way that a sausage machine produces sausage: they will only be devoured. In short, we could say: it is a blind force without concern for what happens to the individual...; infant mortality, maternal mortality, none of these matters...*

(p. 5)

This feeling also extends to the father, who is perceived as "... *an instrument in the progress of existence. I use the word existence*", Bion emphasizes,

> ... *but I'm trying to describe something which has no human characteristics. Thus, from this point of view, it may be that the father, again, is a slave to this same power, then these little rules about incest, etc., don't matter. (...) If the father submits to that force, he will, unhesitatingly, seduce his daughter, and will seduce her into producing more babies. It is almost like: more causes, more*

babies, more bees, more plants, and more people; but very indifferent to what
happens to the people or to the individual plants.

(p. 5)

Bion finally completes the cycle of his reasoning, including the manifestation of
this conflict in the transference: "... *fear that the analyst could be just another one*
of these objects slave to this force – or, alternatively, that the analyst could also
be involved in a hopeless war for individual existence, against this massive force"
(p. 5/6).

Philosophical foundations

Bion's reflections on the case direct us to what Sartre describes in his philosophical
novel *"Nausea"*. I consider this clinical material and Bion's approach to be an excellent illustration of the Sartrean conception that existence precedes essence and,
while essence is still not developed in the mind of the subject, life is a void without
form. This is what the patient refers to when she says she is afraid *"of being unable*
to stop something – which she doesn't know what it is, but still can kill her" (p. 1).
Kill her mind, her thinking. There is a significant parallel with Sartre's comment:
"I'm afraid of what will be born and take possession of me. (...) I would like to see
clearly in me before it is too late" (Sartre, 1938, p. 18).

In the novel, the protagonist, Roquentin – paralyzed in front of a chestnut tree
that sucks the sap of the earth in the task of simply existing without having the
slightest consciousness of its life – wonders about the inhabitants of the city where
he lives. Individuals who drag about in their existence without reflecting on an
essence that would have to be built and conquered. For Bion, this is precisely
the anguish of this eighteen-year-old girl: the feeling that she is a little person of
no importance, kidnapped by biological powers that despise her as an individual
with her own will. It is moving to feel the sensitivity and attunement of Bion, who
was older than eighty years at the time of the supervision, to this girl terrified by
the threat of becoming a slave to an urgency to perpetuate a life she does not yet
understand. To obey a nature that would discard her as soon as the experiment
was over.

I repeat: in the material of this supervision, I was struck by the convergence with
Sartre's conception – which he made clear a few years later, after publishing *"Be-*
ing and Nothingness" – of existence inevitably preceding essence, and how much
the latter needs to be created by each individual if they are to escape the risk of
living a meaningless life.

At some point in the novel, Roquentin asks himself: *"My existence began to*
worry me seriously. Was I not a simple specter?" (p. 119). At the height of despair,
he records the core of his anguish in what could well be words of the adolescent
presented to Bion: "... *here we sit, all of us, eating and drinking to preserve our*
existence and really there is nothing, nothing, absolutely no reason for existing"
(p. 151).

Further on, Roquentin describes in details the painful insight he had about his life while contemplating the old chestnut trees planted in the streets of the public garden of the city where he lives:

> *They did not want to exist, only they could not help themselves. So they quietly minded their own business; the sap rose up slowly through the structure, half reluctant, and the roots sank slowly into the earth. (...) Every existing thing is born without reason, prolongs itself out of weakness, and dies by chance.*
>
> (p. 178)

Roquentin's final note in the novel, when every attempt to rescue a meaning for his life fails, could serve as an epitaph for the patient's grave in case she ends up being killed by this unknown thing within her:

> *Now, when I say "I," it seems hollow to me. I can't manage to feel myself very well, I am so forgotten. The only real thing left in me is existence that feels it exists. I yawn, lengthily. No one. Antoine Roquentin exists for no one. (...) An abstraction. A pale reflection of myself wavers in my consciousness (...). And suddenly, the "I" pales, pales, and fades out.*
>
> (p. 224)

Combining the Sartrean philosophical side with Bion's psychoanalytic vision, this girl is asking her analyst for help so that the analyst can help her find, before marrying and having children, an essence, a meaning for her life, in anticipation of a force that tends to consume her existence in a meaningless haul. It is this force that she does not want to feed when she refuses to eat claiming aesthetic reasons.

Some approximations with "Beyond the Pleasure Principle"

Before ending my commentary, it occurred to me to seek, in addition to the philosophical roots, the psychoanalytical foundations of Bion's position. This referred me to what Freud said in "*Beyond the Pleasure Principle*" (1920), when he speaks of the immortal germ-plasm of which we are mere vehicles. At the beginning of Chapter VI, recalling the distinction he made between 'ego instincts' and 'sexual instincts', Freud refers to Weismann's ideas in "Über die Dauer des Lebens" (1884). He emphasizes the passage in which the author makes a distinction between the somatic body – "*one portion which is destined to die*" (Freud, 1920, p. 65) – and another part, the germ-plasm – "*which is concerned with the survival of the species, with reproduction*" (Freud, 1920, p. 65). He recalls Weismann's conceptions as a support of his dualistic theory of drives: those that seek to lead the living being to the cessation of stimuli and hence to death, and the sexual drives which are "*perpetually attempting and achieving a renewal of life*" (Freud, 1920, p. 65).

It is ironic that this perpetual tendency to renew life may be related to a blind and meaningless existence when devoid of meaning, stripped of essence. By the way, Freud mentions something that is aligned to what Bion says: "*germ cells would behave in a completely narcissistic way*", demanding "*the activity of life instincts to themselves*" (Freud, 1920, p. 70). In a way, enslaving the subject to their purposes. Any similarity to the ideas by Richard Dawkins in "*The Selfish Gene*" (1976) is not a mere coincidence. I end my commentary with the hope that this adolescent girl had, with the help of her analysis and Bion's vision of her conflict, succeeded in winning the war against these blind forces of existence at any cost.

References

Chuster, Arnaldo (2018). *Comentário feito durante painel realizado na Sociedade Brasileira de Psicanálise de Porto Alegre*. Personal Communication.

Dawkins, Richard (1976). *O gene egoísta*. Rio de Janeiro: Companhia das Letras, 2007.

Freud, Sigmund (1920). *Além do princípio de prazer*. Edição Standard Brasileira das Obras Psicológicas Completas de Sigmund Freud. Rio de Janeiro: Imago Editora Ltda., (20) 1976.

Sartre, Jean-Paul (1938). *A náusea*. Rio de Janeiro: Nova Fronteira, 2011.

Chapter 12

Supervision S24

T: The analyst brings this session, which he calls a *sui generis* situation, because this session happened two months after the treatment with this particular patient was interrupted by the analyst. It was possible to have this session because it was during the Holy Week. The analyst had free time in his schedule, offered an hour to the patient and the patient arrived at this time.

Bion: How long has the patient been coming?

T: Initially, he came for five months and then left on his own initiative – left the treatment. After a year passed, he returned and started again.

Well, the motive that made him give up treatment, after those first five months, was because he had a very severe case of obsessive neurosis. It took him so long to wash his hands, for example, hours, to take a bath, four hours, that when he arrived for his analytical session, there were five minutes left until the end. The motive he (the analyst) suggested for interrupting the treatment for the second time was an agreement that he made with the patient. It was the following: if the patient didn't come for, at least, half an hour of the session until the thirty first of January, then, the analysis wouldn't continue, because, the patient wasn't there. So he thought it was not worthwhile. Since the patient couldn't manage to arrive in time, the treatment was interrupted on January thirty first. He (the analyst) put two conditions after this breaking up of the contract, he told the patient that they could continue treatment once more, if the patient thought he could manage to arrive on time to, at least, have a thirty-minute session – this was one of the conditions.

Would you like to speak about it?

Bion: Well, I think that I would be doubtful about that, because then, the patient may play with these thirty-five minutes, or whatever it is. It seems to me to be easier to say, right at the beginning, to a patient: *"Well, if I had a vacancy, I shall want to see you, so many times a week and I would like you to conform to my holiday arrangements"*. Now then, it leaves the way open that the patient has to take the risk of pleasing the analyst – either

DOI: 10.4324/9781003439233-24

by coming or by not coming – whether they will accept that contract. Because, you can say that you won't charge fees for the time that you are on holiday, but you will expect the patient to pay, if the patient takes time off. In other words, one expects the time that you make available to be paid for – what they do with that time is another matter.

Now, I put it like this because, take the previous patient we've just been hearing about, this patient can say: *"I come regularly, I do the best that I can, I come so many times a week, I do everything"*. But what one can say about this is: it's up to the patient to make such use of the time that he wants to make and for the time being, you will be willing to make *your* time available. In fact, you can't tell the patient what use to make of the session. You can make use of it yourself. You can decide that you will make your time available – that's entirely your own affair. But, you can't say anything about what the patient does with it.

T: Dr. X asks you if it's not something already implicit in the contract of work that both people should work together – that they actually work.

Bion: Well, you think it would be, but it very often isn't. The background of this would be: a patient or a child can believe that the parents have to look after them. But they don't! In fact, that's why you get children who are abandoned. But, I don't think that one wants to appear to enter into a contract, which one can't, in fact, keep. You can try if you get some help from the patient. But, one doesn't want to get edged into this position, in which one has said that they will cure them, or do something for them, whether they can help or not. He may not come, or he may be thirty minutes late, or whatever it is, or he may come, like another patient and say nothing. But that is not something that was really contracted – to help a patient whatever the patient may do – any more than you can contract to bring up a child however hostile or whatever it is, you can try.

T: Dr. X thinks if it's worthwhile to say to the patient: *"You're sacrificing your session"* or *"again, you're sacrificing our session"*. If it's worth it?

Bion: I wouldn't say that myself. I would say that the patient seems to feel that they have so much time and so much money available, that they can afford to spend it in that way.

T: In this session, the first one after the interruption, he came, lay on the couch. When he arrived he was already twenty-five minutes late. There was another condition, which I hadn't time to translate before, it wasn't only that the patient should arrive on time for his sessions, in order to recommence treatment, but that he also should leave the parent's home, because his mother was a person that was beginning to be very hostile to him. It was noticed that, when he lived with other people, he managed to keep his schedules. So, when the patient arrived at the session, he was already living away from home, at a pension. The pension owner was a very neurotic woman that had many difficulties in bringing up her own children. He couldn't use the phone, he couldn't take a long time using the bathroom and his time for doing things – these impossibilities – created an atmosphere of tension between himself and the pension owner.

One of the examples he gives is: he had some milk that he wanted to heat and it would only take a minute. The lady wouldn't allow him to heat up the milk. Both started quarrelling, he insisted on heating the milk because it would only take a minute. So, the lady took a plaster statue and threw it at him. It didn't hit him because he hid away behind something. Then she started to throw a chair at him and he held the foot of the chair. Then, one of the children arrived and made peace between them both. But, the lady told him to go away. So, he went to his room and started packing. But as usual, he was taking a long time to pack. Since he was sent away, after packing his packages, he went down and asked the lady to give him back the money owed for the deposit that he made. Instead of staying the whole month, he only stayed nineteen days. So, he wanted his money – half of his money – back. She told him that she wasn't going to give him the money. She would only give the money back if his parents came. Following this, she took him and put him out in the street. He kept protesting that this was not simply possible because, after all, there was a contract between them and he had paid in advance.

Bion: I mean, what contract would there be? Say, in the childhood or infancy.

T: In a child...?

Bion: Or an infant. How did he pay? It's alright for him to say he paid, he paid his deposit and so on. What deposit did he pay his father or mother? What contract, in other words, is there, in which the parent is bound to bring-up a child?

T: The analyst made a transferential interpretation telling the patient that he was seeing him, the analyst, like this woman, that he had broken the contract, that he now wanted to receive back his money *indenization*.[1] It's not the meaning of giving him back the money, but paying something for breaking the contract.

Bion: Well, one could say: *"What's in the contract with the analysis[2] and the analyst?"* It's not a blood relation at all. He isn't the mother or father and yet, the patient is expecting the analyst to do something, which nobody has done so far!

T: After he made this observation, the patient didn't understand it, so he repeated it and he put something else into what he was repeating. That this was a situation already very known to the patient; that he feels that he's owed by the others, that people must have patience with him, give him attention. He feels that those things are owed to him because he has been ill treated by the mother.

Bion: But they aren't! Nobody, really, owes anybody a happy life or a proper upbringing! The only place where it gets near that is where the patient expects this from a perfect stranger, an analyst, to do something, which nobody else has ever done.

T: Well, he made a relation between what he said... what he was going to say and the fact that the patient had mentioned trying to heat milk. The milk was in two little plastic packages in the refrigerator and it was cold and it brought to his mind the cold breast. So, he told the patient, that the patient felt that he wasn't getting good milk, the milk that his mother gave him.

Bion: Yes. But supposing it was warm, who had warmed it? Whose contract is it to warm it? I draw attention to it because one could, even rationally, one hopes to get some sort of cooperation or assistance from the analysis or the analyst. But, we don't know why this is protective. Where has this patient got this idea from? The only contract one could say, that the analyst enters into is: he will do his best, *not* that he will be successful.

T: Dr. X asks if that wouldn't be the infantile omnipotence, magic, that was put on the figure of the analyst.

Bion: Well, again, that is an analytic theory, which is quite useful. But, one has to consider, again, what it looks like in the analysis. Yet, this is again the difference between *practical analysis* and the *theories of analysis*, because in practical analysis, one is supposed to be able to recognize some of these things that have got these names like transference and all sorts of stuff like that.

T: Dr. X asks if it's not a case of infantile narcissism, in which the child requires all the love that is given.

Bion: Again, the point is: what does it look like in a session?

T: Dr. X is trying to answer the question which was raised: *"Where does the child, the patient, expect the analyst's help from, that the analyst be successful and give him something".*

Bion: The point there is: where does this patient, how does this patient get this idea at all?

T: They are talking about the patient's feeling theory, which is based on the fact that since he was deprived as a baby of the mother's care, he expects to receive it, he has the right to receive it from everybody with whom he has a relation.

Bion: Again, I would say: *"Where does the right come from? Why does any mother love her child? Why does any baby think that the mother/father owes them an education, an upbringing?"* You could draw the patient's attention to this, say: *"You are talking as if you had the experience of a contract, which is entered into on the part of somebody, to give you a happy life. But, we don't know where you got that idea from".*

T: And Doctor X said that the requirements of the patient – there was some feeble discussion that followed that – that the patient required of the analyst something; that the analyst believed that this client felt he expected something in return, because of the many things that the patient felt that the analyst had.

Bion: Who is the analyst in charge of though? It is presumably a father or mother, who expects him to behave according to the accepted rules of the house. We get back to this point: where did this idea come from? The patient, very often, will say all sorts of things about how badly their fathers or mothers are behaving, what bad father or mother they are or were. But then, where does the idea come from: that there is a good father or mother? Where did they get the idea? What one could say is: one could understand why the patient did not expect this from analysis, or have a poor treatment, but it doesn't explain why the patient thinks that he will. I could go further and say: there's an idea here that somebody who'll pay the analyst to be properly analyzed or supervised and all the rest of it... but, is there? Who provides the analyst with the knowledge that he has to have? There's an expectation, but it's very hard to say where this expectation comes from, where this idea comes from. Unless, there was a *mother* who looked after him! There might be! When I say a mother, the actual mother perhaps, or an aunt or uncle, something like that, but he must have got the idea somewhere. There must be some reason why he expects the analyst to be properly equipped.

T: This situation reminds Dr. Y of patients that say that they didn't ask to be born and, since they are in the world, well, they expected the world to take care of them!

Bion: Well, yes! Even in the Constitution of the United States, there's a statement that: *"Every man has a right to be happy"*.

[Lots of laughter]

However, when it comes to our business here, where do patients get this idea: that the analyst will take the trouble to be analyzed, educated, qualified and so on and so forth? Where does he think that the analyst gets the money from? Now, it's because that's a mistaken idea that the analyst has to ask patients to pay. It's not because we are trying to take their money away from them or anything. It's because somebody has to pay for this. In the meantime, this idea that there's a sort of fate or God waiting to put right all the things that go wrong, can be quite a dangerous idea. But this statement which is made: "I didn't ask to be born" is really a complete repudiation... nobody says that they asked to be born. It's a complete repudiation of any responsibility! For one can get the idea: who is, or what is this patient defending himself from here? Because, you can hardly believe that a fetus or baby asks to be born! So, where does the idea come from? This idea, where he has to say: "No, it isn't so". Now, one could say again about that that may be a very unimportant question, we know nothing about it, but there is a question about which we know something: who asked me for analysis? Who asked the analyst to see this patient? Now, if the patient asked for the analysis – and one can make out quite a case from that, one way or the other – then one could also say: who does he expect to pay for it then? Who is to pay for what he asks for?

T: Something occurred to him and he would like to put a question. The patient, wouldn't he be defending himself from the fear of what he will have to pay in turn for receiving a little treatment?

Bion: Yes, and more than that: if he makes good use of the analyst and his experience, then he's really showing that his parents gave him something of which he can make good use of, so, they can't be absolutely bad parents.

T: He thinks that a patient would tend to preserve his theory about the necessity of feeling the parents as hostile... his hostility against the parents.

Bion: It's quite possible. Now this – if that is the case – will continue to something which is the need to go on proving that he has a bad analysis, or if he has good analysis, it shows how badly brought up by his parents he was, because he has to have analysis. Now, this is an example of the kind of thing, which we could then translate into technical terms and we could say: *"This is the sort of thing which is the genesis of* repetition-compulsion, *we have to keep on coming"*. Your patient has got to go on coming, time after time, after time and still having bad analysis! Now, it's very difficult to go the other way and you can go through lectures or anything you like about repetition-compulsion, or even read it in a book – very difficult to recognize the animal when you see it in analysis.

    [After a quite long discussion in Portuguese about what Dr. Bion actually means, the following was said].

P1:   You will see, but in the practice you will not see repetition-compulsion?

Bion: No.

P1:   No, in practice, no!

Bion: No, you will see a person.

P1:   You will see a person!

Bion: You'll see a complicated person. In theory, it's quite useful for us, for example, who want to talk about psychoanalysis – there's no good in it at all in practical analysis. I won't say no good at all, but... very little. Because, it doesn't tell you what that looks like, or what even transference looks like, or countertransference. Those are things, which depend on *experience*. Depend on experience, which makes you discover them for yourself. Then, discover that there may or may not be a name for it. I mentioned this last point because sometimes one may find something for which there is not a suitable name. With this patient of yours, what one knows is that something is shut up in this silence. They can't talk, so there's no way of escape... there's no way at which this *silent object* is able to make a contribution. Now, I suggested: one of the things that a patient can be afraid of, if they stop being silent, it goes straight over to making a frightful noise. Now, this sort of thing matters, because it crops up in so many places. Patients who are unable... who never have drawn, never have played a musical instrument, never have passed an exam. I've had that kind of patient. I've had the sort of patient who has never passed exams and so forth... Then, in analysis, it seems as if one makes it possible for them to dare to do so.

T: When you mentioned that the patient was afraid of breaking the silence and start speaking very much and making noises... Do you mean by this word *"noises"*, speaking silly things?

Bion: Well, certainly they've gone to get the same things that they'd be so afraid of saying silly things, or having somebody that calls it silly, that they wouldn't dare to say anything. You could try this approach to the fact that your patient dare not talk, because of what would happen next, that's the initiating something. After all, one could say even the human race, while they were monkeys who couldn't talk at all, they didn't have anything like that trouble when they turned into people. I heard this said very clearly, not in analysis, not in any of these books, but with a patient who was really illiterate and when he was[3] asked: *"Aren't you afraid of doing this dangerous voyage, this dangerous experiment?"* And his reply was: *"Is man a stone that he should live forever?"*

T: Is man a what?

Bion: A stone. The patient can be somebody who dare not be born and really is born dead. They don't show any signs of life. You will sometimes see a patient who will lie on a couch absolutely passive, as if they were a mummy because they are afraid of what they would initiate.

Notes

1 Indenization is a word used in Portuguese for indemnification, compensation.
2 Dr. Bion said analysis. I think that he must have made a mistake. The correct word must be analysand.
3 Two or three words were missed because someone was coughing.

Supervision S24 commentary

Marta Foster

In commenting on this supervision, I sought to somewhat respond to my restlessness regarding this activity. When I 'listen to' the supervisions, they always make a lot of noise and stimulate me to try to see, through Bion's associations, the way I articulate his theories and technical proposals. From the emotional experiences mobilized in me, I will attempt to transmit to the reader how I 'dreamed' this valuable encounter of the trio patient, analyst, and Wilfred Bion.

It is from this apprehension that I intend to present some ideas that I 'dreamed' from the experience presented in the Supervision, since I understand this exercise as an excellent opportunity to expand our 'analytical listening'.

Initially, my attention turned to Bion's question right at the beginning of the Supervision, as it refers to a specific type of investigation. At that moment, Bion interrupts the report of the analyst to ask: *"How long has the patient been coming?"*

My 'listening' was that Bion's curiosity was directed to knowing how much time later the analyst interrupted the work. I thought about the concept of containment, of negative capability, which Bion often refers to in his work. After how much time together the analyst decides that the work is no longer possible? It appears to me that the analyst did not believe that the work was already happening. This seems to make a difference. Was it after days, months, years? Finally, the reference to this fact conveys a specific 'listening' to the analyst. Somehow, this issue will be present in the experience of this analyst with the patient, of this patient with his analyst, of this analyst with his supervisor. The issue there seems to concern time, and not timing.

The analyst's answer was interesting. He initially refers to the interruption of the analytic work as an initiative of the patient. After that, the restart; then the agreement until January 30th. If the patient continued acting/being that way, the work would be interrupted. Lastly, it seems that the question there was very distressing, a minefield area, in which the tolerability was sensitive. I ask: Was it an agreement or a threat?

Can we think in terms of an agreement, when what is occurring is a symptom? Can the symptom be 'eliminated' or 'modified' by the suggestion?

DOI: 10.4324/9781003439233-25

James Strachey, talking about Freud, says:

[...] but it was the abandonment of hypnotism that expanded even further their understanding (insight) of the mental processes. It revealed the presence of yet another obstacle – the "resistance" of the patients to the treatment, their reluctance to cooperate with their own healing. How should one deal with such reluctance? Should it be suppressed with screams and pushed aside by the suggestion? Or, as in other mental manifestations, be simply investigated?

Freud's choice for this second path took him directly to the unknown world that he would explore his entire life.[1]

When I 'listen' to the question asked by Bion to the analyst, these associations come to my mind. I believe that this knowledge about Freud is present in Bion's thinking, as pointed out by the author Adriana Salvitti in her PhD thesis (USP) *Freud's presence in Bion's thought constructs in the 1950s.*[2]

When Bion says: *It seems to me that it would be easier to say, at the beginning, to the patient: "Well, if I have an opening on my schedule, I want to see you that many times a week, and I would like you to agree with my vacation plans.* (p. 2), what I 'listen' is Bion's suggestion for the analyst to occupy a specific place, *i.e.*, to expose his needs, based on the analyst's methodology. Here, I understand that the question refers to the theories that organize that analyst's practice. When Bion says:

It is the patient's decision to use this time that he wants and, for now, you are ready to make your time available. In fact, you cannot tell the patient what use he should make of the session. You cannot say anything about what the patient does with this time.

There is a technical proposal, made by Bion, that is present in the suggested method, *i.e.*, the role of the analyst is to investigate.

In *Learning from experience*, Bion begins chapter X with a 'pearl' for psychoanalysts and psychoanalysis. He says:

Thanks to the beta-screen, the psychotic patient has a capacity for evoking emotions in the analyst; his associations are the elements of the beta-screen intended to evoke interpretations or other responses which are less related to his need for psycho-analytic interpretation than to his need to produce an emotional involvement.[3]

I 'listen' to this communication by Bion, *Making the best of a bad job.*[4] But for that to occur, the analyst must live experiences of symmetry with his patient. The desired symmetry and the capacity for 'reverie' are possible consequences of the 'tolerability' in the analytic room.

When I study Bion, I 'listen' to him giving us some messages, and this one, which I believe to be present in his 'auspicious' question, is one of them.

From the stance that I seek, *i.e.*, "the place from where Bion would bring his contribution", what I 'listen' to refers to the importance that he gives to the condition of the analyst of waiting for what will emerge from his patient. This is implicit in his famous concept, *without memory, desire, or understanding.*[5] He presents to us the limits to which we are exposed in this difficult task, but there is a visible request, in my opinion, that we should always seek this stance. I think this is implicit in his concepts of alpha function and *reverie*.

Bion's proposal underlines the concept of the patient's 'responsibility' for his analysis, for his life. Bion's stance, therefore, is not that of trying to remove the patient's difficulty, but welcoming and attempting to contain and represent this difficulty. In contrast, in the analyst's stance, we can hear 'traces of superego', which could prevent the patient from expanding his capacity to think. Bion's observations seem aimed at trying to help encourage the growth of the patient's thinking capacity, rather than the 'correction' of the patient's behavior.

I thought about the question asked by Bion in reference to the association of the patient who brought an experience that he had with a person who, apparently, had given him an opportunity, but whom he felt was, in fact, a strict and demanding person who had no consideration for him and who 'only' considered his own interests.

Bion's question was:

> *I mean what contract could there be? Say, in youth or childhood... Or a baby. How did he pay? It is OK for him to say that he paid, that he paid his deposit, and so on. What deposit did he pay to his father and mother? What contract, in other words, is there, in which the father is obliged to create a child?*

I 'dreamed' that Bion's words referred to the present emotional experience, in which the patient feels that the analyst must remain at his disposal, whatever his attitude is. I think that Bion presents aspects from the theory proposed by Klein about voracity, which are found in narcissistic personalities. Bion also presents his proposal in relation to 'transformations in hallucinosis', because the thought of the patient in relation to the analyst has 'hallucinatory' characteristics. In my opinion, he organizes his concept in his statement:

> [...] *But they are not due! No one really owes anyone a happy life or an appropriate upbringing! The only place that comes close to that is where the patient expects, from a perfect stranger, an analyst, to do something no one else has ever done.*

I think that Bion cares about the problem of saturation of the analyst's 'listening', as there could be no doubt about the theory that is present in the patient's communication, but the question is how we can do something that can be useful in this situation.

Many non-verbal and pre-verbal communications – and not only verbal ones – are understood as ways to expel the unbearable. For example, the several hours that the patient spends in the shower, his impossibility to arrive on time to the session.

I ask: Is it possible that this patient could become a thinker for his thoughts? I believe that Bion gives us a technical hint in regards to that when he presents to us what he would say to this patient:

> *You're talking as if you have the experience of a contract that someone joins to give you a happy life. We do not know where you got this idea from!*

I believe that Bion's communication is present in his theory that "we will never like what one day we already did not like" (personal communication from a supervision done by Laertes Ferrão), a concept that is also present in Freud's paper "On narcissism: an introduction".[6] In this sense, in Bion's theoretical thought we see concepts addressed by Freud related to the issues of mnemonic traces and all the associative process. Within this approach, I believe that Bion presents the issues related to the theories of *total transference* (Klein) which, in my opinion, is contained in the concept of 'transformations'. For example, in his statement,

> *Who provides the analyst with the knowledge that he must have? There is an expectation, but it is very difficult to say where this expectation comes from, where this idea comes from. Unless there was a mother who cared for him! It could be! When I say a mother, the real mother, maybe, or an aunt, or uncle, something like that, **but he must have taken this idea from somewhere** (my emphasis). There must be a reason why he expects the analyst to be correctly equipped.*

Bion's reference to the issue of 'responsibility' is present in his proposals, as in his theory of thinking. Proposals such as 'getting in touch', 'acceptance/containment', 'reality at the expense of evasion and hatred towards reality' would all be possibilities of achieving knowledge (+K).

When Bion calls attention to the fact that *it is very difficult to recognize the animal when it is seen in the analysis*, referring to compulsive repetition, I believe that his proposal of possible containment and representation illustrates and reflects his concept of 'projective identification' as a form of primitive communication.

In chapter XII of the book *Learning from experience*, Bion says that the activity that we know as 'thinking' is a way to get rid of accretions of stimuli. He says that in fantasy, we believe omnipotently that it is possible to dissociate these undesirable parts of the personality – even if sometimes valued – and place them in an object, and he alerts us to the fact that when we are under the effect of this omnipotent fantasy we may present behaviors that relate to a counterpart in reality.

When Bion talks about his 'listening' to the clinical situation presented, he allows us to know his theoretical concepts, as well as his technical proposal, which he presents to us:

In practice, it is possible and desirable for the purpose of a beneficial therapy to interpret the facts that support this theory and that this theory explains like no other.[7]

When Bion finalizes his contributions by presenting his proposal *The patient can be someone who does not dare to be born and, in fact, is born dead! He doesn't show any sign of life.* 'I dream' that it is associated to the emotional experience present in this encounter between analyst and patient, in which the analyst fights for his patient to develop resources to finally 'be born'. Like a midwife, the analyst seeks instruments in the Supervision, eager to transform beta elements into alpha elements. Bion's words carry his perception of *someone who does not dare to be born is born dead!*, and presents his hypothesis, *because he is afraid of what would begin.* We could think of these words as a search for a successful language, which I believe attempts to put in motion this 'body-mind', which was 'inert' until then.

Biography

1 Strachey, James. The relationship of studies with psychoanalysis. Text: Studies on hysteria. In S. Freud, *Brazilian Standard Edition of the complete psychological works of Sigmund Freud (1972)*, Rio de Janeiro: Imago.
2 Salvitti, A. (2009). Doctoral thesis (USP). *Presence of Freud in the construction of the thought of Bion in the decade of 50.*
3 Bion, W. (1962). *Learning from experience* (1st ed.). Lanham: Rowman & Littlefield Publishers, Inc. (chapter 10, p. 24).
4 Bion, W. R. (1979). Making the best of a bad job. *Revista Brasileira de Psicanálise*, 13 (4), 467–478.
5 Bion, W. R. (1990). Notes on the memory and the desire. In *Melanie Klein Today*. vol. 2, Ed. Imago, Rio de Janeiro.
6 Freud. S. (1972). Introduction to narcissism. In S. Freud, *Brazilian Standard Edition of the complete psychological works of Sigmund Freud (1914)*, Rio de Janeiro: Imago (chapter II, p. 107).
7 Bion, W. (1962). *Learning de la experiencia* (1st ed.). Buenos Aires: Paidós (chapter XII, p. 67).

Chapter 13

Supervision D7

P1: Do you have any suggestion?

Bion: No, I don't mind, whatever you want to discuss.

P1: I would like to ask a question before the material. I would like to know if you think that the transference may be understood as a matter of memory and desire?

Bion: Umhm… I think that it can be anything, I don't think it matters, because the real point about transference is that it's only a psychoanalytic theory of a link between two people, it's talking about a relationship. Now, in this respect, over and over again, it's not unlike mathematics even, in which the point is the relationship between numbers. So that I think that psychoanalysis is really talking about, not you and me, but us, the relationship between us, that's the important thing. It's not the relationship say, between the breast and the mouth or penis and the vagina but the relationship between the objects.

P1: I beg your pardon?

Bion: The relationship between them. For some reason, this is very difficult I find, for analysts, to realize; although that's all it means; transference simply means the kind of way two people are linked – not what is linked to what, but the fact that they are linked. That is what one is investigating: not A and B but plus: A plus B or A minus B. It's the minus or the plus that one is concerned with.

P1: Yes, but I would like to know if, is that link made based on memory and desire?

Bion: It might be made of anything. That is what you have a chance of seeing in the session. Have you an example? Have you the kind of… incident which would cause you to believe that it is a part of it?

P1: That's only from noticing that everything the patient talks to us is something that expresses his memories or his desires.

Bion: That's good enough, that's good enough. The essential thing about that is: if you wanted to talk… here for example, you can use words like memory and desire… perhaps if you wanted to talk to the patient about it, you could say that to draw attention to it, but what you're trying to draw attention to

DOI: 10.4324/9781003439233-26

is the link between them and what this link is composed of. You'll probably have no trouble about that; it may be the only way in which you can describe the link. But, do you have some further point about this?

P2: We must think... that a relationship between two people is always based on transference?

Bion: Umhm... this is something which is peculiar to psychoanalysts. It's difficult to realize what peculiar people we are, because we are so used to it – our patients aren't. Now it so happens that if you are a psychiatrist or psychoanalyst, that kind of person, then it is quite likely that you can see and hear things which a person who is not can't hear or see. So, when somebody comes to you for analysis it's very easy to forget that they don't... they do not know what you know. One of the peculiarities of having an analysis is that it takes a long time to get over the dramatic effect of analysis, of being analyzed. One is constantly under the impression that one's analyst knows an awful lot about oneself. But what one does not realize: that the patient similarly does not know how much you, as the analyst, know.

P2: In which the problem is saying what the patient knows, I think that our... our... expectation, I don't know how to say it in English, is about what we don't know.

Bion: Yes, that is true. But this, again, is a peculiarity that... the more experienced the analyst is, the more he learns how little he knows, how very important that is: the way in which the patient is not so fortunate is that he does not know how ignorant he is. And patients very often think they know more about psychoanalysis or psychoanalysts or... analysis, than the analyst does. It takes them a long time to discover that they don't. So, in fact, you get a situation in which the patient doesn't know what an awful lot his analyst does know, the analyst may be aware of his gap or his ignorance and so on, but it takes a very long time indeed to learn to discover how little one knows and very difficult to realize what a lot there is to learn.

P1: Do you intend to say that the patient... the patient behaves in that way because of the theories the analyst beams on him?

Bion: We have to talk conversational language and so we use words like: envy, hate, love, affection and so on. Now, the trouble with the patient is that he remembers what these words mean and what he remembers is nonsense. So, if I were the patient, I could say to you: *"Oh, yes, I've heard all this: I know about envy and hate and so on. I'm not a child. I know it all"*. But it isn't true; in fact, we stir up memory by using language which the patient is used to and he, therefore, thinks that because we use words like envy or hate or love, he knows what we mean, but he doesn't. When any of us who are analysts or with a psychiatric background talk about envy, for example, we have to use that word but we know something about what envy is; that is the real thing of which the name envy is just a word.

P1:   Do you mean that we know intellectually what the meaning or the conceptualization of envy is, but not the feeling? He doesn't... the patient, the patient does not feel envy.

Bion: Well, he may ...

P1:   Recognize...

Bion: ...he may, but umhm... he may also know the word envy, but whether he knows what the word is that belongs to that feeling is another matter.

P3:   He doesn't know how it operates, no?

Bion: No.

P3:   That's the question!

Bion: No, he can identify himself with the person who has that feeling and he can identify himself with the person that knows that word, but they're not really related. There is not a relationship between those two things. It's only in the consulting room where the analyst has a chance of pointing out:

> *This feeling that you have got is the thing about which you use this word envy, but when you are using the word envy, you don't know what it feels like and when you are having the feeling, you don't know what it's name is.*

P3:   It is more difficult in the schizophrenic patients who... speaking between... it's like speaking... the space and the time and it's difficult to feel what they think about.

Bion: Umhm... this term, this schizophrenic patient, is a convenient way of attaching a name to what I call a constant conjunction: a whole mass of experiences. Now, we borrowed that word from the psychiatrists. It's quite useful to us in a very crude and rough kind of way. But, it wouldn't take a psychoanalyst long to discover that the patient, who you say is schizophrenic, it doesn't really mean anything much, compared with that patient. A name may be very useful if... for example here we want to talk about a patient, it's very convenient to say: *"Well, it's a schizophrenic patient or a schizoid patient"*, some phrase of that kind, but after that we're concerned with details. The analyst is concerned with a microscopic view of that situation, for which the language is, at best, macroscopic.

P2:   That's why the microscopic point of view we can... I think we can never observe what the patient is feeling but what he is feeling only he can... I don't know if I can say, know.

Bion: Umhm...

P2:   His envy is not the same as my envy or like another one's envy and I must, I think, I must present for him... for himself that what he is feeling but I don't know what he is feeling. I don't know if I understand.

Bion: But, again, it's very easy because all the time we are brought face to face with our ignorance. That's something which we've got used to recognizing, our ignorance. It's very difficult to appreciate that, ignorant as we are, we know much more than the patient. So, as a bunch of people, we know very little but a lot more than the patient knows and when any one of us says – envy – we are using a word which has not got the meaning which it has to the patient.

P1:   It's a moral violence? It's a kind of moral violence against the patient?

Bion: Umhm…

P1:   Moral is violence, moral is equal to violence. I…

Bion: Well…

P1:   Constant conjunction, schizophrenic…

     [Two or three words are blurred]
     …is moral violence?

Bion: I don't know because you are… if you are talking about a patient that you've seen for any length of time you know, or even if it's only three sessions, then you already have very great fund of experience.

P1:   We know much more about our patients, when we try to tell something to our patients, we are doing some kind of moral violence to him.

Bion: That is right!! If the patient's cooperating, if the patient cooperates and gives the analyst a chance to give interpretations, then the patient, like the analyst, is colluding to commit an outrage on the patient. Now, in physical medicine, this is tolerably easy to understand; one re-appreciates[1] that although you give your patient an anesthetic and the patient therefore does not feel or know about the assault that's made, the surgeon knows that if he operates on the patient, as operated surgically, he is assaulting, he is assaulting, physically assaulting the patient.

P1:   And mentally either!

Bion: Now?

P1:   Too!

Bion: That's much more difficult. That's much more difficult, because I can say this patient's name is Smith, well, it may be, but I can't say this patient's mind is Smith. That depends on thinking that his skin, his physiological make up, shows you the boundaries of his personality and character. I don't think that's true. So you have got a great difficulty there, which is: that we have to use the language of physical medicine to talk about something which is not physical at all. Now, some of the schizophrenic patients can feel that. That makes it… what makes it difficult, where you can get a psychotic patient, it's quite reasonable according to our categorization, to call him a psychotic, but it isn't only what that patient doesn't know, but what he does know.

P1:   You mean, if we use colloquial language, conversational language, toward a schizophrenic or a psychotic, a psychotic, his way of symbolization could express our conversational… our conversational language, our conversational words, in that… in his way of grasping the meaning.

Bion: Erh... no, I wouldn't agree about that from my experience, but this is a matter which is of the upmost importance and I don't want you to think that my experience is superior to yours or anybody else's – this will never be solved except by analysis.

P1: I thought... I thought that I was quoting you.

Bion: Yes, I know, but I'd like to elaborate this a bit.

P1: In your exhibition about the symbolization of the so-called incapacity of the psychotic or schizophrenic to symbolize and the peculiar way the schizophrenic or psychotic has to... to symbolize.

Bion: I don't think he does it. Let me... let me talk about this a minute. A symbol depends on... you can form symbols, we organize, form symbols, but what this consists of, if you look at it is: bringing together two very different things and seeing the resemblance between them. In short, the peculiarity of the symbol is that it involves bringing two ideas together and making a third idea. Now, that I don't think, certain patients can do. I think that certain patients may appear to be able to do it – they can do the language in a way which sounds like it's got the ordinary meaning, but it hasn't. I don't think that they are able to bring two things together in that way. If you ask me: *"What way?"* I would say: in a way which gives rise to... erh... well, to use a verbal expression: a thought generator or if you were using mathematical language, a number generator. The important thing about this is: both, number and generator, meaning by generator something that is generated. Definitely it's got this kind of sexual meaning and we can know that, but I don't think the patient is able to do that. So that, when the patient, say, has what he calls a dream, I think that the analyst needs to be a person who doesn't bother about this thing called a dream, but makes up his own mind as to whether it's a dream or not. For example, the patient says: *"I had a dream last right"* – this is somebody who doesn't have dreams but he said that happened – why? I don't know... it... it looks like progress in analysis; what it is, is another matter. He says: *"I was sitting next to the driver of the motor bus, I put out my hand to show that we were going to turn right. My arm dropped off and I could see it lying on the ground"*. No free association, nothing, that's a simple fact. Now, you and I might think that this is psychic reality or a psychic fact, but to the patient it's a fact, that's all. It's a simple fact.

P2: A concrete fact!

P1: A real fact!

Bion: Yes, it doesn't matter that it happened when he was supposedly asleep, or anything happened when he was supposedly awake. There are no free associations, so that from the analytic point of view, one can't use that queer dream. It's got no free associations... it's got no dimension, got none of the qualities which make it available for analytical interpretation.

P1: You mean that we really should await, should wait for years until... for days and weeks and months?

Bion: I don't think you can ever say that, because one doesn't know that one's got years or months or even hours available, there's… one of the peculiarities of this business is that we just do not know whether the patient can afford either the time or money to come to us and for how long.

P1: I should respect the fact told by him to me: *"And I saw my arm drop to the floor"*.

Bion: Right! You can see it lying on the green grass.

P1: For me as a layman or a psychoanalyst this is a delusion.

Bion: Well, it may be quite convenient for you to call it that and quite convenient for us that you call it that, because we probably are familiar with that sort of language.

P1: I … I didn't use this… this positive conjunction, the delusion, the words, because of my ignorance of what… of what could be the meaning of his telling me… *"My arm was lying on the floor"*.

Bion: Yeah. Now this word seems to me to be leaving out of account what language this patient is talking and I don't know who's going to find that out, except psychoanalysts. I certainly don't believe that anybody else is; if we don't, nobody else will. But, there's no reason why we shouldn't debate it here. Well, here we've got… after all, we've got a certain amount of language available, which we all can more or less understand. But not in that consulting room and with that particular patient. For example? Supposing I were to say… well as I am saying: *"This is not what I call a dream. This is not what I would call a delusion, this is not what I would call a hallucination"*. Alright, then, what would I call it? I don't know. I don't know what to call it because I don't think that a name exists and this is the other trouble: that as psychoanalysts, we have got to invent the language that has to be spoken as we go along. It's rather like being in the position of an astronomer like Galileo, who has got to make a telescope, before he can observe the stars that he thinks behave in a particular way.

P1: On the grid – can you categorize this, my arm – I saw my arm lying on the floor.

Bion: No. Well, the grid is a very bad and very inferior instrument – it's the best I can do, but it's a bad one. Now, this brings me to this point: it's like a ruler. A ruler is not a theory, but it is made of theories, it's an instrument; and you may or may not be able to use the instrument… to measure, say inches or millimeters or meters by it, for what that's worth, or it might be a watch which you can use to mark the passage of time – assuming that there is such a thing. So, with regards to the grid, I'd say at this point: *"Yes, I would be prepared to try to categorize this… more or less, more or less"*. In other words: I strongly suspect that it could be argued that this does not belong to thought at all, but it may also be on the border, so that I could say that it may be a beta element – which means nothing – or I can say: it's an alpha element – which also means nothing – it's simply an artificial instrument which is useful for talking about it.

P1:   But...

Bion: Yes?

P1:   Understanding this material, understanding this... as the patient says like this: *"We can interpret this in such way, if I will point you the way, you will cut my arm".*

Bion: Now, I would be suspicious about that, although I might have to say just what you've said, because we should be using articulate speech, which is capable of articulation and which is capable of articulating a verbal vocabulary. For example, it will be capable of saying: *"Terrific efficiency. My father is terrifically efficient".* Now, that sounds alright, but by this time I would begin to suspect that it's not good enough to call this patient schizophrenic: that's a macroscopical view; bringing the psychoanalytic microscope to bear, I strongly suspect that the statement *"terrific efficiency"* or *"terrifying efficiency"* which is what I've heard you... is in fact a construct and it is in fact synthetic, in which efficiency depends on something which isn't said in it, but which comes from terrible; and terrible doesn't mean terrible because it's got a component which comes from efficiency. It's a synthesis of terrible efficiency. Now I don't know what this is, but I don't think that it is articulate communication: I suspect that it might be analogous to ideogrammatic speech. In other words, that *this so-called dream is a verbal transformation of visual imagery.*

P1:   There is no thought... there isn't any kind of thinking beneath these words, these ideograms, do you think that?

Bion: Yes.

P1:   No kind of thinking?

Bion: No, I do think so. I do think there's a kind of thinking, but that is... this is just a hunch, a theory of mine, that I think that as psychoanalysts we might find out the underlying... an underlying pattern. Were you?

P2:   Is it possible the sign of language to show some kind of intention to hide the truth... about himself?

Bion: That's... let's take something relatively simple, like Chinese, where you've got a whole lot of ideograms and supposing that a Chinese were to write a letter here or write it on the board; now, when it's written on the board, does that man or woman think from up downwards, from left to right or from right to left? I don't know, but it is not articulate speech, it's ideogrammatic speech.

P1:   Ideogrammatic?

Bion: Yes, and I doubt whether the Chinese grammar and Chinese vocabulary would get us very far...

P1:   They have nearly 400 symbols.

Bion: Yes.

P1:   These... each one has several meanings and the combination of the several ideograms has been... I asked you, I suppose you do not know Chinese?

Bion: No.

P1:   I asked you… this is a kind of symbol, known to the Chinese, not to us.

Bion: Well, I'm not sure it's a symbol or not.

P1:   How could they communicate?

Bion: I don't know, but I think, I think that there must be some sort of valence because if you… you know the common garden story which is said that; what is the property of zinc? Well, zinc combined with sulfuric acid, these two, water and so on, that's not a property, that is a relationship, if you could say that they were animate, then zinc has a personality which can, as it were, have a relationship with sulfuric acid and it is possible in the physical world to talk about various molecules and say that there are some which are available for combination so that you can get a sort of end result which is of salt and water.

P1:   I like very much this example in your book, in your book – Transformations – and the beginning of the process of thought, of thinking, as a kind… in the beta elements, if there is some elements like you put the beta elements, you… you… your… you assume that there should be some traces of thought previous to these beta elements that you do not consider thought and the example of the glass of water with the sulfuric acid and the… sulfate.

Bion: Well, I'll put it a little bit differently because I would say that I have a kind of psychoanalytic prejudice. I have a kind of psychoanalytic preconception. Now, this prejudice leads me to suppose that there is such a thing as transference, but it's a theory. It doesn't mean that the theory is wrong, but it doesn't mean that the theory is right. It's just a theory and theories are neither right nor wrong, they may be useful or not useful.

[By the sound, it seems that a break is taken]

Bion: I don't…?

P1:   We are doing an experience, we are making an experience, we are trying to discover, we are trying to go into.

Bion: Yes, yes, but unfortunately so many psychoanalysts think that the apparatus is available. Now, I don't think that the apparatus is available, is available. Now coffee is what we want!

P1:   Well…

Bion: Well, shall we go on just the same so as not to lose any time? Hum… and I think our unfortunate position is that without any apparatus while this patient is talking or mercifully perhaps is silent, we have to produce an instrument, which will cope with this situation and the question would be: suppose that I think, that I could say something to the patient, what am I to do? Am I to talk, which would be the case with me, conversational English to him, or conversational whatever the languages that he talks, and if not that, what is psychoanalytic language?

P1:   Psychoanalytic language is a language which goes on inside the psychoanalyst, in the inner world of the psychoanalyst, in the psychoanalyst's inside only, do you mean that, do you mean that?

Bion: No, no. I mean here we've got a chance because we've all had certain training and experience and so forth, so we can try to communicate. But supposing there we've got a schizophrenic, or what we call a schizoid patient, what then? What language can we invent here and now which would make it possible to say something to him, in a language that he would understand?

P1:   And this language would be right more than transference language, it is usable for the patient.

Bion: Well, I have a strong suspicion that classical psychoanalysis – without bothering what that is – is not anything like advanced enough to deal with that or really to describe the situation which we want to deal with; in other words, to use a model: you cannot take five oranges away from three and, indeed, in order to do that you'll have to invent negative numbers. Now, when you have invented negative numbers, you've also got to invent or enlarge the area in which... which is bigger in which to use that language; so that classical psychoanalysis, classical psychoanalytic theories and the classical area in which we are accustomed to be – the analytic situation and all that – in which we use these interpretations, that has got to be altered as well.

P1:   May I ask you a personal question?

Bion: Yes!

P1:   Do you sometimes work in a different way, different from the classical way – not using transference, for example, in some situations?

Bion: I depart from it with extreme reluctance and don't like doing so. I don't think it's good enough, but I don't know anything better, but I'm sure it isn't good enough.

P1:   But isn't it a way of making some research?

Bion: Oh, I think so, I think so, but I do think that anybody who's gazed on this analytic work has not only got to do the research, but has got to make them do that well. You've got to make your lens, you've got to make your retorts, you've got to make all this apparatus, mental apparatus, with which to do it and you've got to increase the space. Now at last, at last, the mathematicians have actually woken up slightly. I say this, because I think there's a great danger of psychoanalysts thinking that the physical scientists, quite rightly, are very impressive; their theories are very impressive and therefore they must know a lot what psychoanalysts don't know. I don't believe it and I think it would be fatal to assume that the physicists can teach us anything about scientific method, which they assume will suit us, it won't. So, every one of us... the next patient we see, has not only got to try to use such intuition that we've got, but also has got to invent the apparatus with which to do it.

P1:   You did this when you used negative numbers and analogies...

Bion: Yes.

P1: ...about the preconception of the great. There are negative numbers and positive numbers below.

Bion: Yes, yes. Well, I go further in this way and suggest that one enlarges the space in which to exercise our work, by considering that there is a sort of scale borrowed from sensuous experiences – I mean by that the experience which is available to the senses.

P1: Only this psychoanalysis you are going to do in this way?

Bion: Yes. Now, I also want to suggest that as well as this, there is sensuous, infra-sensuous and ultra-sensuous, and this space has got to be increased to provide the room for the analyst who's seeing a schizophrenic patient.

P1: You call the space?

Bion: For convenience, it's again... using... it's using the same language, it's using again falling back on borrowing language from the sensuous world, but there again, after all, language, I think, has been invented at least as much in order to mislead and deceive one's enemies, as in order to communicate with one's friends, and it is very difficult to use a language, which may well be well adapted for lying and deception and evasion, for purposes of approximation to the truth.

P1: Do you think languages were made for this sense?

Bion: Yes.

P2: A person for... form another one.

Bion: Or to attack?

P1: Or to attack.

Bion: Yes.

P1: And how...

Bion: But this again is something that only we can find out, I don't think anybody else is going to. If psychoanalysts don't do it, I don't think anybody else will be able to do it.

P1: That's a matter of... of fear about communication?

Bion: Umhm... I think that the... I'd like to change the words a bit and say: the human animal, like all animal life, does not like the unknown. So, when confronted with the unknown, the human animal, like all other animals, has both curiosity and fear stimulated and you've got this situation in which curiosity has to be exercised, while the person is afraid, or in the example of the gentleman I spoke of last night, the important thing is: that he goes on thinking, while he's being attacked. The analyst and the analysand are easily mislead into thinking that it's easy to do analysis – it's just talking, that's all and how easy that is!! But it isn't!!! Because in fact, that emotional situation in the office, in the consulting room, is a paradoxical one: it both stirs up curiosity – the analyst is curious about the patient, the patient is curious about this body, who doesn't know what – and both are afraid of that part of it, which is unknown. So, at once, the temptation is to say: *"Oh, he is just Smith!"* and that ends where his skin ends; the boundary of

	it is his skin, because when it comes to the mind, I don't believe it's true, when it comes to the personality, I don't believe it's true.

P2:   You think there are no limitations?

Bion: I don't know what they are. I don't know where the boundary is to be drawn – if there is a boundary.

P2:   But there is a beginning.

Bion: I can see that we are dealing with a kind of expanding universe and every time we give an interpretation, we expand it still further; but whether the expansion is going faster than our interpretations or not, I don't know. It's rather like the astronomer, who is able to make advances into the central field of sight by aid of telescopes and all the rest of it, but that has reached a point in which the double effect, for example, betrays the fact that this has already gone beyond the range of sight and that something has been done in the way of dragging in the x-rays and the... the really very long range wireless waves, to be able to see still further; but whether the distance from here to the limits of x-ray keeps pace with this further expansion, is another matter.

P2:   But in that case of the words and the fear of the unknown we, in the consulting room, may, may have not... may not be anxious because we believe that we can talk, but if we are aware that we are feeling, we are experiencing feelings, we began to be anxious.

Bion: Well and even so, one strong suspicion is that the anxiety is not unlike a dream, it's a relatively tolerable description of something much more frightening. We'll have to think of some different phrase like *"nameless dread"* or some expression of that kind which is again synthetic; it depends on not *dread*, not *nameless* but on the two of them. So I think that the analyst is quite within – well, I don't know what to call it – but normal, if he is frightened.

P2:   By the fact that he's...

Bion: Of what he is doing, of his investigation. But, one hopes that the analyst will be tough enough to put up with that. It's not simple... it's not easy like something... like trying to climb Everest or anything of that sort, because that's relatively physically perceptible. But we are dealing with something which is not physically perceptible.

P2:   It's just answering your question, we are... X was asking if that fear is conscious... if we, the patient are aware, is aware?

P3:   It's a feeling, actual feeling. When you are working...

Bion: Yes, yes.

P3:   How can you describe it, if you can; I don't know.

Bion: You can't, because I think I can say something about I and you, but the moment I'm able to say something about I and you, or you and I, it turns into I and it and you and it – that's quite different.

P3:   Because of the it is neutral? I don't know, I don't know!

Bion: It's, It's restricted, it's restrictive. You've broken up this relationship which is unrestrictive, which is boundless, which is you and I or I and you.
I suppose we'll have to end.

P3: Yes.

Bion: Yes, right.

Note

1 Translator's Note: On the tape Dr. Bion says: *"Reappreciates"*, I could not find this word in a dictionary even in the unabridged Webster. I think that Dr. Bion was emphasizing the word appreciate or he mispronounced it.

Supervision D7 commentary

Aldo Luiz Duarte

Facing a text produced as a result of an encounter with Bion is always a unique experience because of the huge challenge such an encounter represents.

Supervision D7 begins with Participant 1 asking Bion for a suggestion on where to start; to which Bion answers that he does not care, giving the impression that he is actually indifferent to where one begins. The Participant thus suggests beginning with a question: can transference be understood as a matter of desire and memory? Bion answers that transference is merely a psychoanalytic theory of a link between two people, and that when one speaks of transference one is speaking of relationships in the strictest mathematical sense of the term.

One may think that first of all Bion is setting the tone for the conversation – that he will try to move away as much as possible from the sensorial during this entire dialogue, as a helmsman doing his best effort to steer the ship in the ideal direction of the caesura represented by this relationship 'between'. In other words, the question may be related not to the presence of desire and memory, but rather with keeping away from them as much as possible.

But the question remains: what is transference for Bion?

"Transference simply means the way by which two people are linked, and this is what is being investigated", he says. He continues to show and to stress the importance of the issue of the language we are using, and ponders if the patient is capable of understanding it. This leads us to the question of what it is that Bion really understands as "transference", and how much this understanding has to do with what we usually want to convey when using this term.

I have been concerned with this issue, for two reasons. One has to do with a study group. After trying to study transference for a while, we found such a variety of terms and definitions in the literature that we were at a loss on how to proceed.

In addition, I have been following the work of Arnaldo Chuster in Rio de Janeiro, which includes a view of transference in Bion that is seldom described in the psychoanalytic literature; one exception is the work (which I will also discuss later on) authored by Dr. Junqueira de Mattos. In both these authors, the notion of transference is intimately related to the idea of transience, movement. Neither mentions the issue of repetition of the past as something inherent to the concept, except for the fact that all which constitutes us in the present is a history of our past, as stated by Maturana,;

DOI: 10.4324/9781003439233-27

but it is not of that past we talk about when thinking of transference as the classic concept of repetition in psychoanalysis. A quick idea of the thoughts on transference expressed by these authors may help us raise some points here. I will not delve into the discussion of the term "transience", used by Freud, which was translated into Portuguese as "transiência" by Dr. Junqueira de Mattos. For the purposes of the present discussion, I will use the terms transience and transitoriness interchangeably.

For Junqueira de Mattos (2001), all human experience – departing from realizations of the two types of human pre-conceptions described by Bion, always unsaturated, leading to a scientific deductive system in the search for a truth that is never reached – is transitory:

> all our ideas are ideas in transit, on the way to something else... thus transference is made up of feelings and ideas in transit, transient feelings, transient ideas that we place/deposit now on the analyst, now on other persons... but which will not stay there forever, it's a crossing...

(free translation)

Even though Freud was concerned with the theme of transience in his article of 1915, in which he establishes a relationship between transience and mourning, it was not Freud but rather Bion who developed the theme of transference as a transient phenomenon. And after the concept proposed by Ogden that an interpretation is always a product of shared creation in the analytic relationship, and if transference and counter-transference are indefinitely and mutually influenced by each other, how could transference be a mere repetition of the past, if it is permanently re-created within the specificities of the analytic relationship? This is the question posed by Junqueira de Mattos.

In his book "A psicanálise dos princípios ético-estéticos: a clínica", Arnaldo Chuster dedicates one chapter – "Transference or caesura?" – to this theme. Chuster starts by emphasizing the banalization of the word 'transference' after it was 'transferred' to common discourse with disregard to Freud's warning of the importance of our being surprised by the concept. Chuster states that for Freud, transference was always a matter of surprise, and, at the start of his work, even a bad surprise (p. 138). However, with time transference shifted from being a surprising phenomenon to being an expected event, whose absence even causes some degree of unsettlingness among analysts, as if something were missing...

Chuster points out that Bion recovers this surprising character of transference, which, "before being a 'persona' intercepted by the language of the link is something unknowable, ineffable, which he [Bion] names 'O', whose movements or evolutions/transformations characterize transference. The latter is then described by the various psychoanalytic theories, but which no theory can strictly define, since it is not something that can be materialized as text. The proof is the permanent insufficiency of all clinical vignettes, no matter their format. Chuster also states that, in spite of the existence of repetition, as mentioned by Freud and Klein, what matters to Bion is that which is new and unknown, reminding us that nothing ever repeats itself in an identical way. The surprise that is reintroduced in psychoanalysis by the term 'caesura' rekindles the "vigor contained in meanings of generating media and creation, creation and transit, occult transit and explicit transit, blindness and perception of unexpected... what emerges with the movement of surprise". Chuster says that when surprise is expected, it does not show up. What appears instead is the matter that is transferred, the content which he says belongs to transference but is not transference *per se*. The Being of the link is changed by the elements that affect transit, and not by that which is transferred. Thus, there would be no transference movement without change from one mental state into another, "it is the thing itself which moves that constitutes transference".

...

I believe that this – the initial dialogue between supervisor and supervisee, before any mention of clinical material – already provides a very rich topic for reflection... Right from the start, Bion shows his introjected model of supervision, which, like his notion of the analytic session, is very different from the model of supervision in which most of us were trained.

Bion spares no efforts to underscore how important it is for the analyst to keep in mind that speaking with a patient is not the same as speaking with another psychoanalyst. This may seem obvious at first; but as the dialogues proceed, it becomes clear that we often talk to the patient using terms that seem to have been, let's say, "incorporated by use", especially common words such as 'envy', 'hate', 'hallucination', among others. He continuously underscores, more than we usually do, the importance of the particular meaning of such words for the patient, which may be different than the meaning we have in mind. Even considering that we are currently much more attuned to this fact, it is never too much to reinforce the importance of this aspect to Bion.

At some point in the text we have a dream, or, one could say, a supposed dream: "I was in the bus and although I wasn't driving, I held out my arm to indicate that the driver was going to turn. My arm fell off and I saw it lying on the ground".

As the participants resort to psychoanalytic theory to discuss the dream, Bion seems to imply that trying to stick to language is useless. He speaks as if he were trying to leave language behind, to go beyond, to focus on movement more than on eventual meanings that might be statically attributed to the material (dream) which, by the way, was proposed by Bion himself. It is as if the void of associations suggested to him an idea of death. Even the most classically obvious aspect of the dream, which is that of castration (as many of us would be tempted to interpret), seems to be avoided, surfacing through the expression "my father is terribly efficient" with emphasis placed not on 'terribly' and much less on 'efficient', but rather on a synthesis of these terms. Even then, Bion does not see this 'dream' as articulated communication, but instead as something analogous to ideogramic discourse, that is, a transformation of visual images herein falsely denominated 'dream'. Yes, I do understand that this 'falsely' means to him that we are not yet in the presence of what he, Bion, understands as 'dreaming'. Rather, we are in the presence of thoughts that have not yet been thought out (dreamed), and thus as dreams they could only be 'false'... (I ask myself at this point if what he calls a false dream would be a thought without a thinker. I think the answer is yes).

Another colleague from Rio de Janeiro, Renato Avzaradel (2005), begins a work titled "Ideograma e formação de significado" with the following statement: "The concept of ideogram has become since Bion fundamentally important for the understanding of various psychoanalytic developments, in relation to dreams, pictorial language, and thought". He then provides a long and consistent description of how enriching the Chinese language can actually be for us. "The transformation of ideogramic thoughts, through the transformation of visual images into verbal ideograms, into verbal Aristotelian language, that is, language with subject-verb-complement, allows thoughts to be thought out" (free translation). But not before that. The ideogram would be the scaffold for verbal thought.

In 1959, Bion (1992) asked himself whether it would be possible to "get nearer to describing what alpha does". He answers his own question as follows:

> it [alpha] pays attention to the sense impression. But in order to do this the impression must be made durable. It must be transformed so that it is suitable for storage and recall. In short, it has to be submitted to alpha activity, and that is impossible unless durability is conferred on the impression and is itself a part of the process by which durability is conferred. The impression must be ideogrammaticized. That is to say, if the experience is a pain, the psyche must have a visual image of rubbing an elbow, or a tearful face, or some such. But now there enter a new feature depending on whether the Pleasure-Pain or the Reality principle is dominant. If the Reality principle is dominant, then the object of the ideogram will be to make the experience suitable for storage and recall; if the Pleasure-Pain principle is dominant, the tendency will be to have as the object of the ideogram its value as an excretable object.
>
> (p. 64)

I believe that this is the point Bion has in mind when he questions whether the ideogram is or is not a symbol for that patient at that specific moment. He goes on:

> let's consider something relatively simple, like Chinese, in which you have a large number of ideograms, and suppose a Chinese would write a character here or write it on the blackboard; now, when it is written on the blackboard, does the man or woman think top down, or left to right, or right to left? I don't know, but it is not articulated discourse, it is ideogramic discourse.
>
> (p. 9)

It is not dreamed discourse.

It might be asked: is the existence of an ideogram that does not express a thought the equivalent to an unthought thought?

It should be considered that each Chinese ideogram has only one and always the same meaning. Therefore an ideogram drawn on a blackboard is just an ideogram drawn on the blackboard, and that's it. Could it be that when Bion asks if that man or woman thinks top down or right to left he enters the dream and frees the ideogram from its single meaning, so that it can now be dreamed?

The importance of ideogrammaticization as an initial step in the genesis of thought has been considered by many authors, even before Bion. Junqueira Filho (2005) reminds us that as early as 1937 Ella Sharpe brought up this subject by suggesting that the laws of poetic phraseology and those of dream formation originated from the same unconscious sources, leading to the recognition of the dream as the key to the storage of memory and experience. Bion picks up the theme in 1957, Money Kyrle in 1968. Still according to Junqueira Fillho, the storage power of the ideogram resides not in images, but rather on the bonding links that articulate the images: once dreamed, the emotional experiences (stored in the unconscious as ideograms) become the links, the elements that will be mobilized when the psyche needs to produce a verbal thought.

It may be noted that this theme permeates various fields and authors in our culture. I will only cite two such situations that seem to be intimately related with what I said earlier and which, in my opinion, support the ideas described by Bion.

The first comes from Russian movie maker Sergei Eisenstein in an essay dated 1929 and entitled "The cinematographic principle and the ideogram". In that work, while discussing what cinematographic montage is, Eisenstein shows how in Japanese writing the combination of two simple hieroglyphics into a more complex set (the huei-i, that is, 'copulative' hieroglyphs), formed by two belonging to the simpler series

is to be regarded not as their sum, but as their product, i.e., as a value of another dimension, another degree; each, separately, corresponds to an object, to a fact, but their combination corresponds to a concept. From separate hieroglyphs has been fused – the ideogram. By the combination of two 'depictables' is achieved the representation of something that is graphically undepictable.

Thus, Eisenstein compares the process of movie montage to the construction of ideograms.

Parallel to that I would like to cite another moment in which these ideas emerged with great force: the Dada movement in the early 20th century. It is interesting to note that while Eisenstein talked about montage as 'collision' or 'conflict' more than as 'chain', Andre Breton and his Dadaist colleagues talked about 'surprise' and 'disorientation' in the juxtaposition of objects in their art. The value of the image is at the service of the "beauty of the sparkle it produces", they said. "It is not the object itself that lends value to a work of art; it is a certain disposition, combination or positioning of the objects that confers this value…".

Some sentences linked to the Dada movement cannot go unnoticed… such as "many works produced by Dadaism were not preserved in material terms, and survived only as a state of mind that refuses to leave a legacy that is not that of reflection". Or else: "Each generation will have to discover its own means of rebellion and create its image". "There cannot be a more explicit act of faith in the possibility of humans than their capacity for creation" (Cancel, 2004).

Would these concept-sentences sound strange to a group familiar with the ideas of Wilfred Bion?

... And I realize that we are in the terrain of realization. A seminar by Chuster (2010) comes to my mind, in which the first pre-conception phase was discussed: it would occur in the unborn mind, in the primordial mind. Its realization at this initial stage would depend on the mother's body rhythms. Olfactory, auditive, tactile, movement rhythms... the mother waking up, moving, her peristaltic rhythm, all this being perceived by the proto-mental mind as rhythms... a state which, going through the caesura represented by the alpha function, could make us think about the construction of the first imagination, the radical (root-like) imagination. This imagination would lead to the opening of 'windows' capable of receiving the 'landscape' in which the first images are glimpsed (constructed on that spot, not pre-existing); the feelings of orality, anality, etc., that would constitute conceptions, always unsaturated, that would function as new pre-conceptions; and all of this in the direction of the formation of an imagination proper. Thus, the unconscious is inside and in the movement itself.

Bion said that "Like an elephant pursuing a tiger the conscious is lumbering after the unconscious. In such situation psychoanalysis is just a stripe of the tiger".... The less memory and desire, the greater the possibility for the new. And this causes much anxiety. Perhaps an anxiety that is similar to that which was transmitted to me when I read this experience lived by our colleagues so many years ago.

References

Avzaradel, R. (2005): *Linguagem e construção do pensamento*. São Paulo. Casa do Psicólogo.

Bion, W.R. (1992): *Cogitações*. Rio de Janeiro. Imago.

Cancel, L.R. (2004): *Curadoria no Brasil da Exposição "Sonhando de olhos abertos: Dadá e o Surrealismo"*. Catálogo. São Paulo. Instituto Tomie Ohtake.

Chuster, A. et alii (2003): *A Psicanálise: dos princípios ético-estéticos à clínica*. Vol. II. Rio de Janeiro. Companhia de Freud Editora.

Chuster, A. (2010): *Seminário Clínico no Instituto Wilfred Bion*. Porto Alegre. Não publicado.

Eisenstein, S. (1929): "O principio cinematográfico e o ideograma". In: *Ideograma – lógica, poesia e linguagem*. Haroldo de Campos. São Paulo. Editora da Universidade de São Paulo. 1977.

Junqueira Filho, L.C. (2005): "Da esfinge ao oráculo". In: *Linguagem e construção do pensamento*. São Paulo. Casa do Psicólogo.

Junqueira Mattos, J.A. (2001): "Transferência e Contratransferência como fatores da transiência". In: *Rev. Bras. Psicanál.*, vol. 35(2): 335–338, 2001.

Money-Kyrle, R. (1968): "On Cognitive Development". In: *Int. J. Psycoan.*, vol. 49: 691–698. Apud Junqueira Filho, Luis (2005) acima citado.

Rustin, M. (2008): "A estética psicanalítica revisitada à luz da contribuição de Meltzer". In: *Trabalho apresentado no Encontro Internacional "O Pensamento Vivo de Donald Meltzer"*, São Paulo, SBPSP, 29 a 31 de agosto de 2008.

Index

Note: Page numbers followed by "n" denote endnotes.